DOCTOR BUSINESS

Hal Alpiar

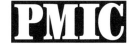

Library of Congress Cataloging-in-Publication Data

Alpiar, Hal, 1941-
      Doctor Business : what they don't tell you in med school or practice / Hal Alpiar.
            p. cm.
      ISBN 1-57066-003-4
      1. Medicine--Practice. I. Title.
      [DNLM: 1. Practice Management, Medical. 2. Economics, Medical. 3. Personal Satisfaction.
      W 80 A457d 1994]
      R728.A394 1994
      610'.68--dc20
      DNLM/DLC
      for Library of Congress
                                                                                   94-3563
                                                                                     CIP

ISBN 1-57066-003-4

PMIC (Practice Management Information Corporation)
4727 Wilshire Boulevard
Los Angeles, CA 90010

THE HOUSE CALL

Of course my mother and father raved about him.

Three or four times a year, he would drive from the next town in his shiny old "woody" station wagon and trudge up two flights of steep, dingy apartment stairs with his bulging black bag to examine or treat my brother and me at home.

I think the reason my folks always greeted him so ebulliently is that he performed this service for a kitchen table pileup of three or four scraped-together, crumpled dollar bills and odd pocket change...plus a cup of coffee and (if it was cold or late) a shot of Dad's whiskey.

I remember standing in front of him, shivering, with my pants down around my ankles, and a little silver, glass thermometer with a red ball on the end stuck into my butt. I remember his sweaty forehead and pudgy fingers. And all kinds of icy cold metal stuff sliding around my chest and back, poking into my ears and nose. I always sneezed. He always frowned and said, "Aha!" or "Hmmmmm."

Actually, I knew from the very first moment of his very first visit, when he turned away from me to mumble something to my parents about not letting me drink my milk until <u>after</u> I ate all the food on my plate, that Dr. Kahn was definitely...<u>not</u> my friend.

ABOUT THE AUTHOR

Hal Alpiar was born in 1941 in New Rochelle, New York, the first of two sons, to an Armenian immigrant father and a first-generation Irish-American mother. The family lived in a tiny, third-floor, walk-up apartment bordering the railroad tracks in otherwise wealthy Larchmont, New York.

From the age of 14, Alpiar worked 40+ hours per week in a variety of jobs, including selling pots and pans door to door to help earn a degree in marketing and philosophy from Iona College.

In his first full-time job (after graduating from college), as a $7500-per-year direct mail copywriter with publishing giant Prentice Hall, he was responsible for creating newsletter subscription and renewal appeal letters targeting doctors and dentists. During this time, he commuted 100 miles a day to attend night school and earn an MBA degree in management and marketing from Long Island University. Alpiar has also completed course work for an MA in human development, and graduated from the 4A's (American Association of Advertising Agencies) Institute for Advanced Advertising Studies in New York, New York, and from the New School for Entrepreneurs in Tarrytown, New York.

Alpiar held management and creative positions with several New York advertising agencies, including Foote, Cone, Belding, Young & Rubicam, and Wells, Rich, Greene. During this time he co-wrote the famous Armour Hot Dog jingle, and created and supervised major media ad campaigns for pharmaceutical companies such as Plough, Dorsey Laboratories-Sandoz, and Bristol-Meyers.

In the field of public relations, Alpiar served briefly as director of public relations for the Pharmaceutical Society of the State of New York, and as marketing manager and editorial review board member for Guidance Associates, Inc., the educational audio/visual and film division of publisher Harcourt Brace Jovanovich, Inc.

While at Guidance Associates, Alpiar accepted a part-time teaching position at Pace University in Pleasantville, New York. Following two years at Pace, he applied for, and was accepted to fill, two concurrent full-time positions (as assistant professor of business and as director of the cooperative education career development program) at Ocean County College in Toms River, New Jersey. He received honors for innovative teaching techniques at both Pace University and Ocean County College.

While at Ocean County College, he also initiated and conducted Gestalt therapy-style group "coaching" sessions, for students and staff, focusing on personal and professional growth and development. These private group meetings, composed of rotating memberships, became so successful that they continued uninterrupted, twice a week, for six years.

The positive results achieved by group participants, and by participants in private industry management training programs Alpiar had initiated on behalf of the college, prompted him to resign his administrative post and tenured teaching position to start his own consulting businesses.

In 1978, Alpiar started UNCOLLEGE (to provide nonaccredited college-level courses to the general public that were not being made available through the local college). The combination of high-quality instruction personnel and methods, and an ambitious seven-day-per-week schedule resulted in capacity enrollment levels.

Alpiar later switched educational service gears away from public markets to zero in on management and staff development programs for corporate and small business groups (including healthcare organizations). Experience with these entities provided the framework for the development of his present firm, BUSINESSWORKS Management And Marketing Consultants To The Health Professions, incorporated in 1982 and located in Lakewood, New Jersey.

Alpiar is former editor-in-chief of *Business Talk* magazine and producer, writer, and host of *BUSINESSWORKS On The Air* radio program, broadcast daily for two and a half years out of Asbury Park, New Jersey. He is an occasionally published poet, has published over 100 articles for national and regional business publications on personal, professional, and organizational development strategies, and has edited a career development handbook, *Job Hunter Action Guide*.

Twice the recipient of federal appointments to United States SBA (Small Business Administration) Advisory Councils for his work with entrepreneurship development and management training, he is listed in *Who's Who in New Jersey, Who's Who in Advertising, Who's Who in Industry and Finance, Who's Who in the East, Who's Who in America,* and *Who's Who in the World.*

Alpiar has three grown children: Haley, Christopher, and Melissa. He and his wife, Kathleen, whom he married in 1987, reside on the New Jersey shore and maintain their (BUSINESSWORKS) consulting practice together.

BUSINESSWORKS specializes in management strategy and implementation for all types of medical practices and healthcare and wellness organizations, and in all levels of medical, health, and healthcare marketing, advertising, and patient/client relationship development.

BUSINESSWORKS clients have typically experienced annual increases in revenues and patient flow in excess of 30%.

DISCLAIMER

This publication is designed to provide accurate and authoritative information in regard to the subject matter covered. It is sold with the understanding that the publisher and author are not engaged in rendering legal, accounting, or other professional service. If professional, personal or other expert assistance is required, the services of a competent professional should be sought. Though all of the information contained herein has been carefully researched and checked for accuracy and completeness, neither the author nor the publisher accept any responsibility or liability with regard to errors, omissions, misuse, or misinterpretation.

DEDICATION

*This book is dedicated to Melissa Monica Alpiar,
my profoundly retarded daughter,
and her wonderful caregivers at
Richmond Children's Center
in Yonkers, New York.*

CONTENTS

ACKNOWLEDGEMENTS

With special thanks for the sea of support and encouragement from my best friend — my loving, talented, self-sacrificing wife and business partner, Kathleen. She brings joy to my heart every hour of my life. Her devotion, optimism, intuition, understanding and hard work have made this book a reality. Kathy truly is "the wind beneath my wings."

For the opportunities to listen and observe: Dr. Robert Edelhauser, Dr. Kahn, Dr. E. Tennyson Phillips, Dr. Donna Mutter, Dr. Robert Dennis, Dr. Steven Berkowitz, Dr. Joe Barmakian, Dr. Bob Warren, Dr. Edward L. Hedaya, Dr. Mary-Ellen Rada, Dr. David Morrison, Dr. Joe Buttacavoli, Dr. Inok Kim, Dr. Margaret Lambert-Woolley, Dr. Steve Lenger, Dr. DelAquilla, Dr. Hoffman, Dr. Jeffrey Alpern, Dr. John Penek, Dr. Charles Trad, Dr. Kim Hediger-Wojcik, Dr. Knight, Dr. Rudolph Taddonio, Dr. Leonard Berger, Dr. Sid Baker, Dr. Rick Guzewicz, Dr. Arnold Zimmerman, Dr. Howard Tornopsky, Dr. Gregory Raiport, Dr. Henry Kaessler, Dr. Steve Crawford, Dr. Dennis Cadigan, Dr. Saul Merin, Dr. Ian Blair Fries, Dr. Steve Krasnica, Dr. Jim Neubrander, Dr. Moshe Rothkopf, Dr. Robert Klein, Drs. Bruce and Denise DiDonato, and special thanks to my friend Dr. Roy Mittman for caring and for jumping in. Thanks, too, to all the underrated, hero-nurses who helped along the way!

For all that I learned about myself, about life, about death, and about doctors: Ken Dychtwald, Barry Stevens, Virginia Satir, Elizabeth Kübler-Ross, Shari Able, Brian Tracy, Zig Ziglar, Denis Waitley, Sue Grunenwald, Petrice Flipse DiVanno, Ilana Rubenfeld, Dick Lewis, Ted Barash, Mary Wells, Sal Rubino, Jack Ford, Robert Kennedy, Laraine Abbey, Phil Katzev, Harry Alpiar, Vernetta Alpiar, Wayne Dyer, Betty Springer, Bob Wainwright, John Gribbin, Steve Kern, Roger Holowchak, Mike Slosberg, Carol Kirsimägi, Jim Duffy, Christopher Kennedy Alpiar, Haley Alpiar Murphy, Marian Marshall, Rick Alpiar, The Marshall Family, Ben Buleri, Joe Santucci, Gene Santucci, Wilmot Oliver, Kevin Bousquet, Jeffrey and Lita Greenberg, Ken Peach, John Dziuba, Jay Arrance, Andy Moreland, Joel Geisler, Raymond Massie, and Dan Duffy.

For teaching me the value of diversion, and the true meaning of unsolicited love: my departed golden retrievers, Olie and Captain, and our cocker spaniels, Madigan and Sam.

For their special help: To Pete and Louise, who let me sit quietly in their coffee shop each morning as I wrote and rewrote and edited; to Jim Davis at PMIC for the opportunity to publish *Doctor Business*; to my super editor at PMIC, Gregg Rogers, for prompting, provoking, challenging, and smoothing over my work; and to my good friend, Rabbi Fischel Todd, for the spiritual inspiration and support.

Thank you. Thank you. Thank you.

PREFACE
(FOR DOCTORS)

No matter what type of doctor you are (or are working to become), and regardless of age, specialization, experience, training, organization/ hospital/university/agency, managed care or partnership affiliation, or length of time in practice, odds are you've devoted *so* much of your life (or will devote so much of your life) to learning about how to deal with other people, that large chunks of your self have become lost, or sidetracked, along the way.

Chances are also that your tendencies toward self-sacrifice, self--neglect and self-abuse have undermined parts of your personal life and limited your ability to increase revenues and patient flow.

Even in the face of major healthcare reforms, *Doctor Business* can be the opportunity of your lifetime.

Your adherence to the personal and professional growth and development strategies, and to the "Quiet Marketing" tactics that *Doctor Business* advocates, will enable you to realize a significant increase in your group or private practice revenues and patient flow, an increase that you should begin to notice within weeks of reading this book and implementing its principles.

In that same period, you may also expect to achieve a happier, healthier, more fulfilling, and more productive personal life. You will feel and behave more confidently, and you will be more in control of your self and your own feelings than ever before.

Doctors locked into managed care organizations who think they need to do nothing to stimulate numbers (because patient and revenue flow is essentially determined by contractual agreements), will discover that they stand to benefit from *Doctor Business* in substantially different but equally meaningful ways. This will be particularly true with the advent of healthcare reform, whatever its final form and content, as many of these same doctors find themselves applying what they learn in markedly more competitive environments than they may have originally anticipated, or bargained for.

In either case, this is not a book of magic formulas. There are no seven powerful principals. There is no promise of greatness by following fourteen hocus pocus steps, or by dashing off a dozen daily deeds. *Doctor*

Business is simply an approach to thinking and doing that works. It is an approach filled with offerings to pick and choose from, offerings that will stir your creative juices, and that have been proven effective many times over with doctors and other healthcare professionals of nearly every conceivable type and description.

Doctor Business is based on successful front-line experiences with thousands of business executives, and more than twenty years' worth of doctor and healthcare consulting in the areas of self-development and management and marketing.

The efficacy of this book, and your being satisfied with it, is based on you having an open mind, a commitment to and a desire for improvement, a willingness to let *Doctor Business* be your personal coach, and an active participation on your part — pen in hand — as you read.

In the process of writing *Doctor Business*, it quickly became clear that there is, to paraphrase an old saying, no way to please all of the doctors all of the time. And though much had to be left unsaid due to time and space limitations, *Doctor Business* nonetheless sets forth the trail markers for a less-traveled pathway that most assuredly will produce better results than the majority of well-worn business or personal advice roads most doctors tend to follow. Use this book as your guide.

Over one hundred doctors have read all or part of this book during its preparation, or somehow contributed to the manuscript itself. Without exception, all have endorsed the objectives of the book and the personal, first-hand-experienced, arm-around-the-shoulder-while-kicking-butt approach to presenting ideas and information. Each doctor has acknowledged learning something of value. Each has found something to laugh or smile about in what they read, and each reported a sense of anxiousness to read whatever parts they hadn't yet seen. Finally, each doctor encouraged the birth of *Doctor Business*.

By following *Doctor Business* through to the end, you'll find you have nothing to lose, everything to gain, and that it will be an absolutely splendid journey of doctoring and business revelations filled with positive and constructive thoughts. I would like to express my deepest appreciation for each reader/contributor's time, attention, interest, and support.

PREFACE
(FOR NONDOCTORS)

If you live with a doctor, or work with or for a doctor, if you sell to doctors, if doctors are clients or customers of yours, if you are the patient, friend, neighbor or business associate of a doctor, if you hate doctors or love doctors, you need to be doggedly in pursuit of understanding their behavioral quirks and figuring out what makes them tick, in order to get to know them better, and in order to more fully gain their trust, respect and cooperation.

This is not to suggest that doctors are all the same. Of course they're not. But doctors do appear to have more high level socioeconomic and educational life values, more common interests, more shared characteristics, and a deeper sense of camaraderie than practically any other non-sports professional group. Doctors are truly a breed apart. They have different ways of thinking about time and space and people and things and events. They have different ways of behaving and of taking action. They have different points of view about government, healthcare, politics, education, money, family, business, life and death, and themselves, than most other non-doctor people in the world.

No one has ever written a book about doctors for doctors to help doctors be more successful as businesspeople by helping them be more successful as human beings. Neither has anyone ever written a book that attempts to help those whose lives are regularly touched by doctors to better understand, in simple terms, what being in the business of doctoring is really all about.

In aiming to fill both of these vacuums, I wrote this book with three purposes in mind:

1) To help doctors understand that by reaching inside to learn more about themselves, and by using more of what they learn, they can create higher levels of personal happiness and professional success than they ever dreamed possible;

2) To help all those who come into direct contact with doctors to better understand and appreciate doctors' lifestyle uniqueness, the paradoxical insensitivities they often exhibit in dealing with others, and the overload of stress factors they're subjected to day after day and night after night;

3) To help doctors' families, friends, associates, employees and patients grasp more fully and relate more readily to the unscientific imperfections of the art of doctoring, to break down the myths of doctor omnipotence, and to help people learn how to deal more directly and in a more critically informed manner with almost every type of doctor in almost every type of environment.

If those were my purposes and objectives in writing *Doctor Business*, what, then, were my reasons? I wrote *Doctor Business* to have more impact in the world than I was capable of as a teacher, coach, consultant, marketer, speaker or trainer. I did it because doctors need help with learning how to be more of themselves. I wrote *Doctor Business* because I could see by the consulting style I've developed over the years, that I was able to help; that doctors responded to me and the approaches I used. What do I do that's so different from anyone else? Probably nothing, except that I don't put doctors on pedestals. I don't imagine halos around their heads. I talk with them, not at them or up or down to them. I only call them "doctor" in front of other people, but always show them respect as human beings. I don't "pull punches" when something difficult needs to be said. I listen very carefully and very actively. I understand their stresses and value their pursuits. I seek always to provide them with a strong dose of reality and a reliable sense of direction.

I believe *Doctor Business* provides a strong dose of reality and a reliable sense of direction. Your focus as a reader is intentionally pointed into the present (vs. past and future). You are guided into discovery channels, and coached toward developing immediate, practical ways to make the most of doctor lifestyles, doctor relationships, doctor careers... and doctor business.

Whether you are a doctor or a non-doctor, *Doctor Business* will help you be better prepared for the greatest series of opportunities you have ever had in your life. It all begins tomorrow, and will repeat itself with each and every sunrise.

Dear Doctors

You are not really competing among yourselves.

You are competing to break through old customs, beliefs, images and fears ... you are competing for your share of life.

After 20 years of working with you, I can assure you that "History" (yours) is "in the making" as you read this.

With great appreciation for who you are becoming

Hal Alpiar

P.S. Regardless of your specialty, and whether you're a physician, dentist, chiropractor, psychologist, psychiatrist, podiatrist, et al, if you have the title "Doctor," you also have the need for help with Patient, Staff and family management, and with making marketing functions work to increase revenues and Patient flow... now.

This book will help you ... now. Hal

I

A WAKE-UP CALL

Doctorpreneurs

Doctoring has changed. Whatever it was that got you where you are is no longer good enough to keep you there. In fact, odds are that something about your profession will be vastly different by the time you wake up tomorrow morning, assuming, that is, that you sleep tonight. Acknowledging that there are always exceptions to the range of characteristics commonly shared, doctors in general are very much like entrepreneurs. Both are agents of change. To ensure continued growth, both have a need to make things happen (vs. waiting for "the action" to come to them), to be progressive thinkers and doers, and to respond quickly to marketplace initiatives and technological advancements.

Successful doctors and entrepreneurs both tend to be self-empowering, quick decision makers with fairly strong delegation skills. Both exercise commanding (often domineering) egos. Both are motivated by the desire for personal achievement and financial gain, as well as a deep sense of things spiritual. Both take reasonable risks.

As a doctor, you also — like an entrepreneur — spend enormous amounts of direct and indirect energy persuading others to have confidence in your judgement and trust in your skills. The similarities are important.

But the differences are equally important (if not more so) to the similarities. While entrepreneurs market products, services, and ideas, you market healing, relief, care, wellness, and hope. Failed entrepreneurial ventures can cost a great deal of money and leave broken dreams behind. But your failures can result in more than the loss of money and/or professional dreams; your failures can leave behind scarred and broken bodies. Sometimes a failure on your part can cost someone their life.

One particularly telling characteristic common to highly successful doctors and highly successful entrepreneurs is that both instinctively begin their journey toward improvement by focusing first on themselves. Show me a multimillionaire who's not constantly seeking to learn more about him- or herself, and I'll show you an inheritance beneficiary or a lottery winner. Truly self-made, successful people are perpetual, tenacious students of their own thoughts, feelings and behaviors.

Until you know what *really* makes you tick, and continue to learn more every day, you will never be able to feel completely successful because you will never be able to manage your self and your psychological environment with maximum effectiveness. If you can't manage what's inside you, you'll never be able to manage what's outside you, such as other people and the often trying circumstances of your profession.

Did you ever wish you could feel like "TGIM" (instead of "TGIF") for a change and be happier to be starting out a new week than to be ending an old one? How often have you thought you'd like to have greater influence over your front desk person, a partner, associate, difficult Patient, a spouse or lover, or your children?

The more you can learn about your *self* and how you think and act and respond to different stimuli, the closer you get to making things happen... like motivating, inspiring, and relating more productively to others, instead of just watching other people's parades pass you by, or "wishing" for fantasized results.

My Doctor, The Artist

Doctoring today is at least as much an art as it is a science. And a great artist doesn't study art. A great artist studies him- or herself. Only by knowing what's inside, can a person truly express those traits, characteristics, and feelings artistically, on the outside.

Artistry in medicine has a lot to do with how you "come across" to others. Being aware of *how* you are perceived is the first step to painting more meaningful pictures, to building greater authenticity in your behavior, and to generating greater numbers of new Patients in your practice.

Just by understanding *how* others absorb and mentally "process" your actions and words, you begin to gain greater self-expression and you learn to exercise increased self-control. This increased self-control (and the awareness of how you're perceived) will actually set the stage for you to strengthen your position and influence with associates, Patients, staff, friends, and family.

Almost as quickly as you experience this sense of strengthening (and without even trying), you should begin to generate increased revenues and

Patient flow on a permanent, ongoing basis. It will simply happen. And just as effortlessly, you will also begin to achieve a new level of physical closeness and a higher level of consciousness and spirituality with those you love.

How you walk, talk, sit, stand, speak, listen, gesture, touch, and treat everyone around you every day makes a statement to others about who you really are. It also sets the tone for staff and associate behavior. Frowns, smiles, temper tantrums and back pats are all contagious. They are also all *choices*. You *choose* your own behavior.

Consider, for example, that no one can "make" you angry or upset; you "choose" to feel that as a reaction to someone else's behavior.

Being conscious of this distinction won't necessarily eliminate upset feelings, but it will serve to prompt a *response* instead of a *reaction*. A response implies control, and a conscious and mature method of thinking and acting. A reaction implies an impetuous, immature nature; one who acts before thinking. Choosing a response will help you move through upsetting situations more quickly, and have fewer battle scars to show for it.

Choosing Partial Integrity is Like Choosing Partial Pregnancy

Because you're a doctor, you are also automatically considered to be some form of surrogate parent to everyone you come in contact with. People don't merely "notice" your choice of behavior, they *microscopically examine* your every word and action. Every move you make, you make on stage, in the spotlights. But that doesn't mean you need to start acting like someone you're not. It does mean you need to be (as Thoreau once urged) "forever on the alert."

How many times have you seen a television camera scan through a professional baseball team's dugout, only to settle on a closeup of a player picking his nose or scratching his crotch, oblivious to the scrutiny his actions are receiving. The people around you every day scan their mental cameras to take closeups of you. They see the *real* you, even as you might seek to represent yourself differently. And they "see" when you least expect anyone to be looking.

I know a highly prominent surgeon with *the* perfectly dressed, tanned, and manicured body. He has *the* perfectly behaved (and noticeably subservient) family. They live in *the* perfectly located $2 million estate.

He drives *the* perfectly stylish expensive car. His public behavior seems to have been scripted for him by a cadre of etiquette book authors.

Stepping back from his trying-to-impress-others existence, however, one doesn't have to be a psychoanalyst to see that he is an extremely unhappy and unfulfilled human being. His lifestyle and manner of presentation are so dull that he could easily pass for a human doornail.

Take a look in his private "closet," the most personal inner circle of his existence. Stacks of "girlie" magazines fill the top shelves of his private office bathroom. Sensationalist talk shows on the radio of his stylish, expensive car fill his travels between hospitals. A few too many vodkas fill his bloodstream before bedtime every evening, especially for someone who's going to be doing major surgery after breakfast the next morning (God forbid he be called in the middle of the night to perform an emergency procedure). And, behind closed doors, he tops it all off with endless streams of sexist and off-color jokes, and worse, a daily routine of female staff fanny-patting and skirt-lifting, especially with those staff members he knows fear unemployment.

So what's wrong with that? Doesn't everybody do it?

Everything. No.

Every single move a doctor makes, even that which he supposes is made privately, is actually made in public. Lack of privacy comes with the territory.

This doctor's staff view him as two-faced, insincere and pretentious. They feel sorry for his intimidated Patients, but long ago stopped trying to cover up for his "personality defects." Some members of his staff actually give his more disgruntled Patients whispered referrals to competing practices. His sexual harassment victims may be afraid to speak up, but their silent torture and desire for retribution is starting to take its toll in the many unconscious ways they undermine his credibility and dilute his Patient flow.

How could he think that none of his staff would use his bathroom and notice his magazines when he's away, that none of them would see what station his car radio is always tuned to, that none of them would hear his tasteless jokes or notice the recurring hangovers, that no one would be offended by his sexual advances?

How could he think that the image these "personal defects" project could possibly fail to give rise to doubts about his values, and ultimately, his medical skills? *How* could he think his staff members wouldn't move on to other jobs (often with competing practices), and bring their perceptions of him along to share with others (usually for many years)?

How? How? How? How do doctors get this way to begin with? **Answer:** Medical schools, private practices and group associates ignorantly disregard or purposefully downplay the realities and importance of doctoring *conduct.* Medical schools, private practices, and group associates fail to develop leadership and teamwork skills outside of clinical settings. Doctors simply never learn how important it is to encourage staff people to think and act in terms of "our" Patient instead of "my" Patient, not to mention thinking in terms of Patient instead of patient. Medical schools, private practices and group associates fail to provide the training or experience essential for doctors to understand just how impressionable and sensitive the people are who will work alongside them.

Does this mean you need to be neurotic about your every move? No. It means you need to be more conscious of the moves you make because others already are conscious of those moves. It also means you need to learn how to master things like "presentation skills" and "people skills" for yourself because such realities are not part of standard medical degree studies.

Where There's Smoke...

How laughable the doctor who, as you enter her office unannounced, quickly jumps up from behind her desk with one hand behind her back and a stream of cigarette smoke rising from behind her head. Could she possibly be thinking no one would notice? Even outside her office, with nothing in her hand, could she possibly think no one would smell the smoke in her hair, in her clothes, on her breath? Nonsmokers can smell smoke in paper documents — from three feet away! Just like an overweight fitness instructor, how credible is a doctor who smokes? (In fact, how credible will some perceive the doctor to be whose *staff members* include smokers?)

All day, every day, the image you project is heard and observed and processed and commented on by others. Fairly or not, these images add up to associate, staff, and Patient judgements about how skilled you are. And *that* adds up to Patient referrals...or condemnations. It's your *choice.*

Choosing Death By Thumbtacks

Just as every Patient referral needs to be personally and genuinely acknowledged, so does every Patient complaint, no matter how seemingly frivolous or insignificant. A negative comment must always be taken seriously and responded to immediately. *One rotten apple rots other apples quickly.*

For every complaint voiced (or written), there's said to be a minimum of ten more that go unspoken. Additionally, you can expect that each unhappy Patient will tell at least ten other people about his or her bad experience, and many of those folks will tell even more, on a second and thirdhand (and usually exaggerated) basis.

So, added together, consider that each expression of dissatisfaction with *any* aspect of your services, office or staff, will probably lead to at least 100 negative images of you. Put another way, one negative Patient encounter a week can equal 5,000 negative impressions a year. Can your practice afford numbers like that?

The best time and place to handle complaints is when and where they occur. Make Patient Feedback Forms standard procedure for every office visit. Even when a patient comes every week. Even when a patient comes to see you two or three times in one week. And be sure the staff member responsible for handing out the forms to each Patient makes a "big deal" out of it by emphasizing how important the doctor considers that Patient's opinions to be on that particular day. If the forms are going to be passed out like so many worthless leaflets at the intersection of Times Square and 42nd Street, don't bother to waste the time and expense of printing them, and think again about how committed you really are to reviewing and processing the forms. Think again about how committed you really are to boosting Patient volume and revenues.

If you choose for your own (or your staff's) convenience to follow the apathetic path of "Yes, But" or "Maybe Later," you are choosing to prevent these critical evaluations from ever being planned, printed, distributed, collected, and seriously considered. You are essentially choosing to not learn from your Patients.

The forms must be collected from Patients *before* they leave your office. Studies show that very few people will return forms like this by mail or on return visits. The forms must be reviewed regularly (daily, perhaps five minutes at the end of the day, when possible, or at least once a week — longer than a week makes any warranted response too untimely). And since your Patients are the very source of your livelihood, these forms can also be the single most important source of information about how you're doing, and about what you need to do more of and less of to be truly successful.

By not actively soliciting Patient ideas and opinions, you are electing to remain stagnant. You are literally investing in maintaining the status quo, the easiest, safest, least threatening (and most boring) of all choices. As a result, your practice is destined to die, slowly and painfully, long before its time. You might as well choose death by thumbtacks for yourself. *Working without seeking and valuing feedback is an unconscious choice to not believe in yourself and your own potential.* It's a choice that flies inexplicably in the face of the very same kind of guts and gumption that got you through medical school, internship, and residency.

Ask and Ye Shall Receive

Feedback forms serve other noteworthy purposes. When they are tended to with as much importance as the standard Patient history forms in your practice, the simple act of feedback-form opinion-soliciting will actually short circuit negative comments and even dilute negative thoughts. And, by virtue of how your actual responses chosen are expressed, the wording of those responses can itself squash negativity.

Notice in Figure 1.1 how the phraseology of the questions can minimize the tendency to drag out or exaggerate any negative feelings that might be present. For example, the last choice, "Ridiculously long," in the second question, is phrased in rather extreme terms on purpose. Some who think the wait really *was* "ridiculously long" may not be so quick to actually circle that option for fear of appearing to be too radical (a common resistance factor even on anonymously-submitted survey forms).

The act of circling a seemingly less radical (more civil) option, such as "too long," indirectly serves to tone down the level of upset the Patient may be feeling. And those who do answer "Ridiculously long," will be getting the upset feelings off their chests as they circle the choice and, having been provided a meaningful outlet for expression, are much less likely to carry the upset home with them.

In contrast, those who have no on-the-spot feedback opportunities that a survey form like this provides *will* take their upset feelings home. They'll be prone to tell others that the wait was "ridiculous," perhaps even "forever" or "terrible" or "torturous." In a highly plausible worst-case scenario, they might even tell others, "Don't go there, it's not worth the wait. There's a doctor I know across town who will see you right away. I should have gone there in the first place."

The questions in Figure 1-1 provide valuable feedback. As you

Figure 1-1 front

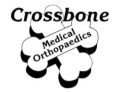

Crossbone

OUR "PLEASE-HELP-US-TO-HELP-YOU" PATIENT SURVEY

(Please circle your best choices for each question)

OFFICE

1. Do you find our (Uptown / Downtown / Midtown / Out-of-town) office to be (clean / attractive / comfortable / average-looking / uncomfortable / messy)?
2. Was your wait for care (appropriate / too long / ridiculously long)?
3. How long did you have to wait before receiving care (less than 15 minutes / 15-30 minutes / longer than 30 minutes / seemed like forever)?
4. Were you greeted in a (friendly / courteous / cold / unfriendly) manner when you entered our office?
5. Were your questions regarding Managed Care, Medicare and insurance claims answered (thoroughly / incompletely / confusingly)?

WHAT CROSSBONE MEDICAL **OFFICE** CHANGES, IF ANY, WOULD YOU SUGGEST?

_____

_____

TELEPHONE

1. When you called our office, did you hear someone who was (friendly / courteous / attentive / cold / unfriendly)?
2. If your call was put on "hold", did we return to you (promptly / after a short delay / after a long delay / never)?
3. Do you feel (satisfied / not satisfied) with the way your calls have been handled?

WHAT CROSSBONE MEDICAL **TELEPHONE** CHANGES, IF ANY, WOULD YOU SUGGEST?

_____

_____

STAFF

1. Do you find our Staff to be (helpful / courteous / attentive / impatient / cold / rude)?
2. Did our Staff answer (all / some / none) of your questions?
3. Did you find the appearance of our Staff to be (appropriate / clean / attractive / just okay / inappropriate / sloppy / dirty)?
4. Compared to other doctor office visits, would you rate our Staff (better than most / average / worse than most)?

WHAT CROSSBONE MEDICAL **STAFF** CHANGES, IF ANY, WOULD YOU SUGGEST?

_____

_____

Figure 1-1 back

DOCTOR

(Dr. Crunch / Dr. Cringe / Dr. Yelp / Dr. Axeblade / Dr. Shatter / Dr. Upchuck)
...Circle names of all Doctors seen during this visit or series of visits.

1. Please rank order, 1-5 (1=most. 2=second, etc.), the five most important reasons you chose a Crossbone Medical Doctor:
   ___ Reputation of Crossbone Medical
   ___ Reputation of individual Doctor (Name):_____
   ___ Referral (Friend / Family / Neighbor / Another Doctor / Lawyer / Service)
   ___ Referral (Coach / Trainer / Teacher / School Nurse / Employer)
   ___ Recall positive advertising message and / or news story
   ___ Convenient office locations Uptown, Downtown, Midtown & Out-of-town
   ___ Association with Major Calamity Medical Center
   ___ Association with Slipshod Hospital
   ___ Provides same day, in-office surgery at Downtown Location
2. Did the Doctor answer (all / some / none) of your questions to your (complete satisfaction / partial satisfaction / dissatisfaction)?
3. Did the Doctor spend (enough / not enough) time with you?
4. Was your (exam / treatment / set of instructions) thorough (Yes / No)?
5. Did the Doctor seem to be (understanding / attentive / disinterested / too busy)?
WHAT CROSSBONE MEDICAL **DOCTOR** CHANGES, IF ANY, WOULD YOU SUGGEST?

_____

GENERAL

1. Will you refer Crossbone Medical Orthopaedics to your friends and family (Yes / No) Why? _____
2. Are you a member of a group or organization that might be interested in having a Doctor or someone from our Staff be a speaker? (Yes / No)
   Who may we contact to make arrangements? _____

WHAT CAN WE DO TO SERVE YOU BETTER?

_____
_____
_____

Thank you for your help. You can be sure your responses will be given priority attention.
We appreciate the opportunity to serve you.
—The Doctors and Staff
Crossbone Medical Orthopaedics

review the responses on the form, be reminded that "professionalism" is not a term that applies singularly to your medical skills. A "good doctor" is someone who is thought of as being easily accessible and possessing professional empathy skills as well as having a strong clinical reputation.

Overheard at the Podiatrist's Office

The following is an actual conversation overheard between four senior citizens sitting in the waiting room. Names have been changed to protect the "innocent."

Senior A: "She's very nice, you know." (Referring to the podiatrist)
Senior B: "Yes, I hear she is. My neighbor's been seeing her regularly for three or four months and says she's very gentle, not like old Doc Cementshoes!"
Senior C: "Do either of you know any good eye doctors? I need new glasses and my sister thinks I might be getting cataracts."
Senior A: "Well (reaching into her pocketbook with a 'I just happen to have' smile spreading across her face), I've always gone to Dr. Blurry, but I cut out this ad (unfolding a piece of newspaper from a zippered pouch) for the new doctor down the street here. It says (as she proudly displays the ad like a kindergartner showing off a finger painting) Dr. Newcomer can do that new laser stuff and he also takes Medicare."
Senior D: "I heard him talk on the radio. And he sponsors my granddaughter's Girl Scout troop. Sara Scuttlebutt told me at the church dinner that he's very friendly. She said he even gives every patient a questionnaire that asks what you think about him and his staff and office, and when you hand it in, you get a fresh flower!"
Senior C: "That sounds like what I need. Someone who will treat me like a person."
Senior B: "I know exactly what you mean. The last eye doctor I went to took two hours to get to me and then acted like I was a truck engine. He didn't even smile once. You'd have thought he was preparing me for life or death surgery, just to get a new lens prescription."
Senior C: "Let me write that number down, that Dr. New-what's-his-name?"
Senior A: "Newcomer. Dr. Newcomer. Here (handing over her ad and smiling, as if the purpose of having cut it out and carried it around had finally been fulfilled). It sounds like you could really use a friendly doctor."

Senior D: "You'd think for all the money they make, these doctors could at least *act* like they care about us as people."
Senior A: "You're darn tootin' they could!"
Senior B: "You can say that again!"
Podiatrist's receptionist: (who has walked out to the waiting Patients from behind her desk and counter) "Thank you for waiting so patiently, folks. Dr. Stepeasy has been tied up on the phone helping another doctor with an emergency, but she'll be with you in just a few minutes. Are all of you okay about waiting? Does anyone need to use the phone?"
Senior A: "No thank you, but you tell the doctor she should take care of the emergency, we can wait, no problem, because you're so nice." (They all nod in agreement.)

The Five P's Principle

By soliciting feedback from your Patients, by showing that you are interested in what they think and how they feel, you are substantially increasing the odds of pleasing more of them more of the time, and Pleased Patients Produce Prospective Patients.

There are many cases of Patient Attitude Surveys being credited with solidifying relations with happy Patients, giving unhappy Patients cause to reconsider the validity of their disenchantment and (by both word of mouth and specific written suggestions provided on the forms) actually increasing referrals of new Patients. There's even additional value in having a survey like this serve as a catalyst for staff development and the improvement of associate relationships.

Rather Than The Rule

When I was a little girl, doctor visits were major events. No matter how much of an emergency was at hand, it was usually obscured by the proclamation that the doctor was on his way. Everyone would scramble around to "pick up the house" and whoever was sick or injured had to be in fresh, clean clothes.

I remember my brother, with what turned out to be a broken arm, crying and writhing in pain as my mother forced him to hurriedly change out of his stained baseball shirt into a clean one as the doctor was pulling his car into our driveway.

And, God forbid, any of us kids should dare to ask the doctor any questions. "Don't bother the man, dear; he's very busy and has to see other people too" (like Santa Claus on Christmas Eve, I used to think). Knowing mother as I did, though, I often wondered if she was merely afraid of having to pay more, based on the number of questions the doctor had to answer.

Anyway, questions or not, he always seemed to have the exact right answers for everything. I used to feel better just to see him walk in the door. He was so warm and friendly. He actually seemed to glow sometimes. All he had to do was touch my hand or shoulder, and I would feel better.

My admiration for him is probably what prompted my parents to prod me into getting my RN Degree. I did. And now, after 20 years of working with doctors, I've only once met another like him, a genuinely warm, caring, human being-type doctor with a cheerful manner and gentle touch. How shameful it is that this has to be the exception rather than the rule.

— A Patient/Nurse

II

THE PERCEPTUAL
PECULIARITIES
OF REALITY

"Fear Tactics" Bring New Patients

It's not enough anymore simply to nod your head and pat someone's hand or shoulder while saying "everything will be alright." To be *genuinely* understanding about someone's pain or discomfort, you need to be sure Patient illnesses or injuries never become so routine that you prevent yourself from imagining how each person feels. Patient distress can never become so routine that you prevent yourself from being nontechnical, straightforward, compassionate, and specific in your personal explanations. Remember:

1) Every single Patient you see is a troubled consumer.

2) Clear communications (to each Patient) are as important for you to provide as your medical skills.

3) Your best source of new Patients is existing and past Patients.

Keep in mind that the majority of Patients who come to you with what are essentially minor ailments are filled with fear. Possibly as many as 90% of Patients are dealing with rational or irrational fears of the unknown, but this fear may not always be easily recognizable. It may be disguised as nervous attempts at humor or giddiness. It may show up as anger, obstinacy, or a macho attitude.

But you can be absolutely certain that fear is always present, and even when it's irrational or the ailment itself is imagined, it all seems very real indeed to the patient. You have to imagine what it's like to be in the Patient's shoes. One good way to do this is to go out (*this weekend*) and rent the movie *The Doctor* starring William Hurt. Watch it twice.

The ability of you and your staff (and the tactics you use) to relieve not only the physical symptoms that prompt Patient visits, but the accompanying fears, whether rational or irrational, will greatly affect Patient decisions to return or not return, and to refer you (or not refer you) to others. Why? Because to each of us, "perceptions" are often considered to be "facts," especially when we can find reinforcement nearby. To put it more concisely (and more poetically), "What we perceive is what we believe."

What Patients perceive about your ability to treat them *and* your ability to soothe their fears, to touch gently, to be empathetic once they've entered your workspace environment — even by telephone — will fully determine the extent to which you get referrals.

A renowned ophthalmologist who specializes in cataract surgery (and often does 30 removal/implants per day) has built much of his reputation among the senior citizen population he caters to by having a full-time, salaried employee designated to do nothing else but (and here's the official written job description): "Give hugs and hand-holdings to waiting, arriving, and departing Patients; bring them snacks and make them feel comfortable and relaxed by the time they see the doctor." The business card title for this employee is "Office Ambassador."

A helpful formula to keep in mind is: **Perceptions + Performance = Referrals**. We only "buy" what we perceive as having value. The need to continuously build and maintain a positive image and reputation is as important to the *immediate* financial success of your practice, as the need to continuously develop and maintain your clinical skills is to your *long-term* financial success. One doctor, representative of the mind-set of many others, acknowledges this thinking as disconcerting:

I've worked my whole career to be able to shut down emotional involvements with patients, to remove myself from their feelings so I can get through the day without ending up as a basket case. You get conditioned early on, you know? I interned at a major city E.R. where we had an unwritten (but strongly-adhered-to) rule that we would only accept 'jumpers' who had fallen two stories or less (which happened about two or three times a week). Anything more than a two-story journey was rerouted to another hospital. You can imagine how quickly I learned to be emotionally uninvolved with patients; '...a three floor jumper? Sorry, that's one floor too many for us. You'll have to take him to Parachutist's General Hospital down the street.' Desensitization is almost a requirement for being a doctor. And now I'm supposed to relate and empathize more in order for my practice to survive and grow?

In his book, *Healing The Wounds — A Physician Looks At His Work* (Pantheon Books, New York, 1985), Dr. David Hilfiker at first rationalizes that clinical detachment takes less time and energy. He then notes, "Not surprisingly, the physician, under the pressures of everyday doctoring, often begins to use this tool of clinical detachment for another purpose: as personal protection...to spare...burning out." Hilfiker points out it's "no accident that the talk of medical personnel is filled with references to people as if they were diseases or parts of the body.

Overheard at the OB/GYN's Office

Doctor: "What have we got in Room A right now?"
Nurse: "Infertility. And Room B still has a first time pelvic waiting."
Doctor: "Did the hysterectomy post-op get here yet?"
Nurse: "That one's running late so we rescheduled it to the end of the day. But the yeast infection just arrived."

"Yes, but that's our way of protecting the privacy of our patients," goes the rebuttal from the doctor. Mrs. Johnson may not want her neighbor, who might be within earshot, to know that she has cervical incompetence, or crabs or whatever. A valid point, except that a lot of departing Patients probably would strain to see or hear who the yeast infection *is* in Room C, and except for the fact that these discussions that reduce Patients to depersonalized body parts and symptoms also take place when there are no Patients around.

Overheard Between Two Orthopaedic Surgeons

The following is an actual car phone conversation overheard between two partners in an orthopaedic surgery practice.

Doctor A: "Don't we have a knee, a wrist, and a couple of ankles hanging around?"
Doctor B: "Yeah, the knee's at the Medical Center. I think the wrist and ankles are at the hospital."
Doctor A: "You want to take the knee?"
Doctor B: "Okay. While I'm there, I'll check out the hip and the hand job."

Doctor A: "Damn! (laughing) You always get the handjobs!"

Detachment for the sake of communicating with other doctors and for the purpose of putting your technical skills to work is acceptable and understood by most Patients. Clinging to a detached attitude when a Patient looks into your eyes, pleading for an answer, or bashfully bows to search the floor for some reassurance, however, is simply not acceptable.

This detachment vs. empathy issue is not some "catch-22-quandry-between-a-rock-and-a-hard-place" situation. By allowing for more intimate levels of understanding to occur, you are creating increased opportunity (for both you and your Patient) to grow. Such allowance is an active choice you can make even now, as you read this.

Mental Exercise

Close your eyes for ten seconds and flash ahead in your mind to the inevitable. See your own dead, lifeless body arriving at the funeral parlor. See your insides being suctioned out via trocar and emptied into a sink en route to the sewer. Then see your corpse being suspended and dunked into embalming fluid. Or, see your body arriving at the crematorium and being placed into the furnace. Or left untreated for burial, and later being eaten by worms, insects, and bacteria, or sharks and marine life if you're buried at sea.

A ten-second flash is usually more than enough to remind yourself that you *are* your body (so is each and every Patient) and that there's more to life, and doctoring, than the aloof, detached dispensing of clinical skills. How much more compassion and understanding can you squeeze into a day? What does it take? How much freer will your spirit be in knowing that you've helped *whole persons* to live or die better, as opposed to simply fixing (or botching) a part of someone's body?

Many doctors are still living in the dark ages when it comes to their attitudes about Patient relations. Management advances may not move quite as rapidly as technological advances, but the notion of providing quick fix "Patient Service" was long ago replaced by the 1980s concept of staying in contact with Patients long enough to check and ensure "Patient Satisfaction." Both of these approaches have been overshadowed by the current emphasis on TQM (Total Quality Management) and what I call "DPR" (Developing Patient Relationships). TQM and DPR both dictate the need for serious, long-term energy investments. *The Patient is essentially viewed as the object of a lifelong relationship that the doctor is responsible for cultivating.*

DPR can be accomplished with an ongoing mix of communications. One-way communications, like newsletter mailings, are most effective when they are interspersed with some two-way efforts, like "How Goes It?" telephone calls by both doctors and staff members. DPR means taking full responsibility to provide ongoing, continuing attentiveness, even when it's not responded to (as is often the case with newsletters and notes).

Postcards For The Edge

Annual (or semiannual) "Checkup Reminder" postcards get dramatically higher numbers of response calls (to schedule appointments) when they are supplemented with intermittent newsletters, occasional seminar invitations, and cheerful, friendly staff reminder phone calls made periodically throughout the year.

One sports medicine client sought to expand its Patient base beyond the market limitations of the few elite, professional athletes catered to in the past. An inexpensive series of monthly educational postcards was created for mailings geared to people engaged in "active lifestyles" (Figure 2-1). To build a targeted mailing list for the postcards, a coupon newspaper ad was used (Figure 2-2). The ad was also reprinted and distributed as a flyer through mailings to coaches, personal trainers, and fitness and aerobics instructors. Additionally, it was used as a handout in the office and at "active lifestyle" area events (like 5 and 10-K runs and community health fairs). Physicians in the practice also made the flyers available at talks, training programs, and team exam sessions. One Little League coaches instructional program run by two of the practice's doctors resulted in 300 coupons returned!

A substantial name, address, and phone number list was compiled of area dance and exercise groups, road race running and cycling participants, weekend athletes, parents of sports-minded children and active young adults who were interested in receiving the free monthly card mailings. The list continues to grow through referrals.

Next, we set up a basic first-aid approach for the type of information pertinent to active lifestyle injuries; one monthly mailing card per injury on topics like Shin Splints, Achilles Tendinitis, Runner's Knee, Tennis Elbow, Ankle Sprain, Heel Spur, Carpal Tunnel Syndrome and Shoulder Bursitis & Tendinitis. Each mailing card focused on "What It Is," "What

Figure 2-1

ACTIVE LIFESTYLE INJURY INFORMATION CARD SERIES

Tennis elbow

What it is This active-lifestyle injury is an inflammation of the fibrous cord, or tendon, which attaches the forearm muscles to the outside of the elbow. It is a common problem in many racket sports -- hence the name, "Tennis" elbow -- but it also occurs in any activity which requires heavy use of the forearm muscles such as golf, fishing, gardening or using a screwdriver.

What happens When the forearm muscles are used repetitively, the tendon can become overworked and inflamed. The result is pain on the outside of the elbow... often made worse by even the simplest of tasks like shaking hands or picking up a coffee cup.

How to deal with it Treatment consists of resting the forearm muscles. This may require a complete break from the sport or activity involved for a week or two to prevent recurrence. A properly placed tennis elbow strap can also help relieve aggravation of the tendon.

Cold packs on the elbow three or four times a day, twenty minutes at a time, can also help reduce inflammation. A sports doctor can determine the value of oral and injected painkiller drugs, nonsteroidal anti-inflammatory drugs and ultrasound treatment. Once the elbow has calmed down, a program of stretching and strengthening can return the elbow to normal. A gradual return to the activity is recommended.

How to prevent it There are several ways to prevent this often painful condition. Warming-up before engaging in physical work or sports is key to most injury prevention and certainly holds true for tennis elbow. The same stretching and strengthening exercises used for physical therapy are great to loosen up with. Having a racket, golf club or tool with proper grip size and using the proper stroke and leverage are also important.

AMERICANA
Sports Medicine Associates
ON CALL 24 HOURS FOR EMERGENCIES
CALL:1-800-NEW-JOCK

ACTIVE LIFESTYLE INJURY INFORMATION CARD SERIES

Shin splints

What it is Shin splints are a common, painful leg overuse injury. They are characterized by pain in the front and sides of the lower leg that develops and worsens during exercise. The condition is most commonly experienced by runners (joggers, sprinters and distance runners alike) and by aerobic dancers. Shin splints are the result of injured muscles.

What happens The condition can be caused whenever the area where the muscle attaches to the shin bone is put under excessive stress. This may lead to a buildup of pressure in a muscle, inflammation of a tendon, a muscle tear, or inflammation of the outer layer of a bone.

How to deal with it Because it is extremely difficult to differentiate between shin splints and cracked bone or a pinched-off blood supply, it's usually best to consult a sports physician to confirm diagnosis and initiate treatment.

Treatment focuses on reducing the stress along the shin bone. This is accomplished by reducing running or dancing activities until the pain decreases. Exercises may be prescribed to help balance leg muscles. The weak muscles in the shin are strengthened while the strong muscles in the calves are stretched. Some cases may require medications or physical therapy. Full activity can be resumed as symptoms decrease. Recurrent symptoms should be evaluated by a sports doctor because this condition can easily lead to stress fractures.

How to prevent it You must balance your exercise program. Avoid overtraining the calf muscles while ignoring the shins. Muscle imbalance occurs when one muscle overpowers another. Add new routines gradually. Muscles that are tightened by hard exercise are more susceptible to injury. Warm up properly and know when to stop. Pain is a warning signal from your body to your brain telling you to stop.

AMERICANA
Sports Medicine Associates
ON CALL 24 HOURS FOR EMERGENCIES
CALL:1-800-NEW-JOCK

Ankle sprain

What it is One of the most common active-lifestyle injuries, an ankle sprain results when the ankle turns beyond the limits allowed by the surrounding ligaments (tissues which connect the bones). Ligaments naturally stretch but become injured or torn when they are stretched too fast or too far.

What happens Usually occurring on the outer side of the ankle, sprains are often immediately painful, and accompanied by swelling. With a severe sprain, the ankle may even become black and blue. The spectrum of ankle injuries can run from a mild stretch of the connective tissue to a complete rupture of a ligament.

How to deal with it Usually, swelling and pain are *not* the best indicators of how bad the sprain actually is; a visit to the sports doctor and an x-ray is usually recommended.

Full recovery from an ankle sprain requires prompt care and proper treatment. Initially, the treatment of choice (easily remembered by the acronym "RICE") is: Rest, Ice, Compression, Elevation. This stage is followed by gently walking as soon as it feels comfortable -- letting pain be the guide.

Next comes rehabilitative stretching and other exercises -- usually best designed and supervised by a sports physician -- to restore flexibility and strength to the muscles and ligaments around the ankle. Safe return to activities is guided by demonstration of the ability to hop on the toes of the affected foot and to run figure eights or zig-zag without pain.

How to prevent it Preventing ankle injuries requires proper footwear (high-tops preferred), and an exercise routine to stretch and strengthen the ankle.

AMERICANA
Sports Medicine Associates
ON CALL 24 HOURS FOR EMERGENCIES
CALL:1-800-NEW-JOCK

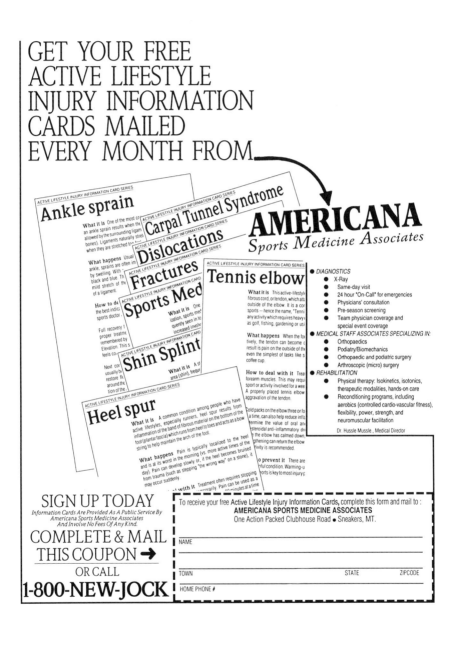

GET YOUR FREE ACTIVE LIFESTYLE INJURY INFORMATION CARDS MAILED EVERY MONTH FROM

AMERICANA *Sports Medicine Associates*

● DIAGNOSTICS
  ● X-Ray
  ● Same-day visit
  ● 24 hour "On-Call" for emergencies
  ● Physicians' consultation
  ● Pre-season screening
  ● Team physician coverage and special event coverage
● MEDICAL STAFF ASSOCIATES SPECIALIZING IN:
  ● Orthopaedics
  ● Podiatry/Biomechanics
  ● Orthopaedic and podiatric surgery
  ● Arthroscopic (micro) surgery
● REHABILITATION
  ● Physical therapy: Isokinetics, isotonics, therapeutic modalities, hands-on care
  ● Reconditioning programs, including aerobics (controlled cardio-vascular fitness), flexibility, power, strength, and neuromuscular facilitation

Dr. Hussle Mussle, Medical Director

SIGN UP TODAY

Information Cards Are Provided As A Public Service By Americana Sports Medicine Associates And Involve No Fees Of Any Kind.

COMPLETE & MAIL THIS COUPON ➜

OR CALL

1-800-NEW-JOCK

To receive your free Active Lifestyle Injury Information Cards, complete this form and mail to:
AMERICANA SPORTS MEDICINE ASSOCIATES
One Action Packed Clubhouse Road ● Sneakers, MT.

NAME

TOWN   STATE   ZIPCODE

HOME PHONE #

Happens," "How To Deal With It," and "How To Prevent It."

A new card was mailed every 30 days, quietly marketing the sports medicine practice's logo, office addresses, and 24-hour emergency phone number. Recipients are encouraged to acquire and keep the complete set in their workout areas or medicine cabinets. Cards double as handouts for individual Patients experiencing an injury that relates to a particular card topic, and as handouts at appropriate doctor presentations (e.g., a talk on Carpal Tunnel Syndrome, or Cycling).

Quality Care Pursuits Outperform Promotional Promise

Of course doctors and staff people who seek to grow a practice must be actively engaged in the daily pursuit of "zero defect" quality care goals. They must do this by staying attentive to the clinical basics and staying in touch with all the latest healthcare advances. Performance failures here will short circuit Patient returns and referrals, and it won't matter how effective your communications pieces or promotional literature (even postcard programs) promise to be.

Doctors and staff people who seek to grow a practice must also be committed to building and maintaining long-term Patient relationships. The sports medicine postcard mailing series that's shown is a good example of one way to do this. Those who don't appreciate how important long-term Patient relations pursuits are will never come to realize their fair share of Patient returns and referrals.

And in case you think this doesn't apply to you because you're not a primary "Repeat Patient" healthcare provider like a GP, OB/GYN, pediatrician, podiatrist, ophthalmologist, dermatologist, physical therapist, family physician, dentist or chiropractor, you're sadly mistaken. Successful doctors, even those with few repeat Patients (e.g., specialists in cardiology and orthopaedics), cultivate and value long term relationships with every Patient. Why? Because, in the end, no matter how infrequently you imagine meeting one Patient's needs, and no matter how massive or powerful your network of referring professionals, the most successful doctors are those who recognize that the greatest number of quality referrals come from satisfied Patients, Patients who feel a "relationship" exists with you, even if they haven't actually seen you in years!

There should never be need to question the investment of any time, money, and energy spent in building Patient relationships. There should never be need to question the value of anything that can be done to improve staff communication skills, and to stimulate increased camaraderie, commitment and trust — the four cornerstones of quality management and DPR management.

Drs. S. Ocrates and P. Lato: A Dialogue

Question: "I'm getting the message that staff communication skills can be improved with increased attention to listening and feedback and simple, straightforward speaking delivery. I also understand that improved communications will help build stronger Patient relations and increased staff productivity. But 'communicating more clearly' can't solve everything. How do I begin to stimulate camaraderie, commitment, and trust among associates and support staff? How do I get people to wake up and abandon the lethargy in which they've become mired?"

Answer: "'Communicating more clearly' won't solve everything by itself, but it can *help* to solve everything. And it can most definitely contribute to increased camaraderie, commitment, and trust among associates and support staff. As for how you begin to build these relations, you begin in the same way you would get a Patient to do these things. To figure out what map you're going to follow and how you're going to get where you're going, you need first to get a true bearing on where you are, then start taking inventory of where you've been."

"Only a conscious review of your past will suffice to establish a strong reference and experience base for setting meaningful new directions. As the recruitment ad heading for a major university's career development program asks: 'How do you get where you're going if you don't know where you're coming from?'"

Take A History

What's the very first thing you do, or have done, to every single first time Patient? Do the same thing to your self. Do it to your practice. Take a history. Do a diagnostic workup. Don't just sit there and read about doing it. Don't imagine doing it. Do it. Would you accept excuses from a Patient? Of course not.

If you choose not to set aside enough "history note-taking" time right now, don't. Get and carry a pocket notebook instead. Jot down your "history" as it occurs to you in bits and pieces — at traffic lights, on elevators, between patients, on bathroom breaks, at your bedside, etc. Or use a cassette recorder for later transcription. You can always scribble in the margins of this book as you're reading. You can also start with the space provided on page 25. (Really. It's okay to mark up this book. It's yours. And your notations and highlights will positively add to your retention — remember your old textbooks?)

If taking this first step is too much hassle, if you think you can gain as much by simply reading this book and not doing the initial workup, or if you think you know enough not to have to bother with doing this written inventory exercise, then there are some things you have to think about: 1) You're probably not ready to begin increasing Patient flow and revenues right now. You may want to pass this book along to someone who is; 2) Consider what your resistant attitude says about your real self. If your attitude is something you would like to change, you can start by simply choosing to change your response to the idea of writing down your history. All you need is a pen.

So pick up your pen and begin *writing*.

Why all the fuss about actually writing? Because by the simple exercise of writing down the historical pluses and the minuses of your professional career experiences, and the high and low spots of your practice, new ideas will begin to surface.

Just by taking this inventory and writing it down, you will start to see some measurable results. You already know the information, but by transferring it out of your head, down your arm, into your hand, and through the pen onto the paper, you are getting it out of your brain! That means less mental clutter in your memory banks. It also means you can begin to take a more organized approach to your sense of business and professional development.

By focusing your mind's energy on you (even on the minimally prescribed basis for intermittent note-taking), you begin a purposeful evaluation process that will raise your consciousness level to a point where you will interact more productively with others.

Let's suppose your staff people have been acting particularly grouchy toward you and/or your Patients lately. How can these same behavioral awareness dynamics help to set up a more pleasant attitude environment? Simple. Just think about smiling more.

When you think a lot about smiling, you tend to smile more. And they're *real* smiles, not the token ones some doctors turn on and off like water faucets depending on which side of the exam room door they happen to be standing. When you smile more, others around you begin to smile more. (Believe it or not, your dentist is not the only one who enjoys seeing teeth framed by upturned lips.) Smiling more on the outside can start you feeling better on the inside. Others will recognize and respond to all this pleasantness with pleasantness in return. Bingo! You start to get more of what you want from others. And it's that simple. You smile more. They smile more. The more smiling there is, the better everyone feels and behaves, the better the Patients will feel about visiting your office, the more you increase your odds for Patient referrals.

Smiling. It's quiet. It's ethical. It's effective. It's less work (you use 12 muscles to smile vs. 103 to frown). It's free. It's the best marketing there is. It must, however, be consistent and sincere. Consistently done, day after day, with a sense of determination, positive attitude interactions (like those represented by more frequent smiling) will, in turn, produce more positive exchanges with others. In very short order, these exchanges can begin to influence Patient flow and revenues. But this is just the beginning. And all you have to do to become a believer is to give it your best shot for three weeks. Three weeks.

Here's some space to get you started. Make some quick notes before you move on.

_____

_____

_____

_____

_____

_____

_____

_____

_____

_____

_____

_____

Overheard Under the Dining Room Table

The following conversation was overheard coming from under the dining room table at a dinner party for four married couples and two of their children. Thirty seconds into dessert and the accompanying standard discussion of diets, the cherubic innocence of three year-old voices, weakly camouflaged behind a conscious attempt to muffle their exchange of comments with loud whispers, wafts upward from under the table...Christopher, and the neighbor's daughter, Annie:

Christopher: (whispering) "I want to."
Annie: (whispering louder) "No, *I* want to. You got to do it last time. I'm putting my clothes back on. It's your turn now."
Christopher: (whispering louder still) "But it's *my* mother's termomadore so I should be."
Annie: (yelling in a whisper): "Too bad! Take off your pants or I'm not playing."
Christopher: (whispering quietly) "Oookay." (Pause. Sound of corduroy rustling.)

Have you ever seen eight adults simultaneously gasp and lift a tablecloth to look under the table? And the spectacle that presented itself? Two naked kids with an assortment of plastic doctor and nurse instruments and one large outdoor "termomadore" that was last seen coming loose from the patio wall.

Annie's Mother: "Hey, you two, what's going on?"
Annie: (sounding disconcerted) "Christopher always wants to be the doctor but he never lets me tell him my problems. He just keeps stickin' the ear and nose thing in my rear and the termomadore in my mouth and makin' tongue noises."
Annie's Father: "What do you mean by 'tongue noises,' Annie?"
Christopher: (as rescuer, offering explanation) "I do the 'tsk-tsk' sounds, you know those clicking noises like Dr. Petey Atrick makes for checkups?"

III

IN YOUR FACE

More thinking space. More writing space. If you're serious about growing your practice, get your pen on the paper. This book can only be your coach. An effective coach will usually elect to use one of three approaches to get you motivated: ignore you, put an arm around you, or get in your face. Your motivational needs have probably been ignored too long, and the first two chapters already "put an arm around you." So, it's time to get in your face: You're nowhere near your potential. Start writing your ideas. Here. Now!

_____

_____

_____

_____

_____

_____

_____

_____

_____

_____

_____

_____

_____

_____

_____

_____

_____

As you think about things and begin to write them down, here's something to be thinking about: *You become what you think about.*

_____

_____

_____

_____

_____

_____

_____

_____

_____

_____

Just as you would probe a Patient about personal family history, be sure to include a section on changes that have occurred with your "professional family" (i.e., partners, business and medical associates, advisors and staff). To get some realistic perspectives of its own unique transitions, view your practice as a separate entity. Make notes about the posture of your practice (as well as your own personal posture) in your professional community. Make notes about how you and your practice "measure up" in your public community.

Take A Lighten-Up Break

Pretend for a moment that you're a cartoonist. If your practice was a cartoon strip or an animated film, what would it be called?

_____

* Who would the star characters be?

_____

* What famous voices would be used for which characters?

___

* Would there be a "good guy" and "bad guy"? Who would be who?

___

* What kind of background music would be featured?

___

* Would the lighting be bright and airy? Dark and gloomy? Romantic and sexy?

___

* Describe the pace of action

___

* Would your production be an award candidate? In which categories?

___

As you continue the process of exploring your own medical history, be sure to note what you recall about the images you think you have both commanded and failed to command. Examining your failures is like asking a new Patient for the cause of a parent's death; it may not always be relevant, but it could shed some critical light on diagnostic issues and patterns.

Finally, and most importantly, take stock of the kinds of impressions you have made with your own personal family and with your closest personal contacts.

As you're writing about each of these considerations and issues, jot down a 1-10 (retrospective) rating to indicate how satisfied you felt with yourself and with others *at the time* they occurred. Then, give each a second rating which indicates how satisfied you feel *now* about each of those circumstances, actions and people. Build in references to when and where you started in practice, on what basis and with whom. Have you relocated since you started? How often? Did each move accommodate your goal-thinking at the time? Are you considering another move? (To expand? Consolidate? Get away?) Are you 100% clear about what you expect a present or planned move to accomplish?

Success Is The Journey, But You Need A Destination

Next, you need to think about goals. Old ones. New ones. And before you run somewhere to throw up because you hate dealing with goals, consider that your (probably) inherent preference for immediate gratification may be prejudicing your response.

Confronted with the subject of goals, most doctors think first of hockey and soccer. Possibly, they think of "treatment" goals, or goals for getting their latest gadget inventions patented. Since, inherently, most doctors seldom think beyond the next hour (especially when they can hire others to plan for them), "goals" have a tendency to be erroneously equated with long-term planning — intangible, unrealistic, distasteful stuff that's better left to nonprofit researchers, corporate lawyers, and tax consultants.

But goals are not limited to Patients and patents. And goals and long-term planning are not synonymous. Most doctors ignore or avoid goals because they don't understand what you are about to read concerning how to set goals and how to use them: *Goal-setting is critical to your own personal and professional success. You become what you think about.*

Stumblebums

One client practice's struggles have been highlighted by unanimous refusal of the partners to acknowledge the need for a strategic plan. Of the four doctors involved, one says he sees the practice becoming a major research resource; another sees it becoming a revenue-focused business entity; a third espouses the need to maintain the status quo (of a benevolent healthcare service without regard for Patient's ability to pay), with no changes. Dr. "Status Quo" is purposefully committed and, in fact, outright obstinate about keeping everything as is. The fourth refuses to assert herself or commit to any direction. There is no direction. There is no leadership. There are no plans. The practice stumbles aimlessly along, day to day. And not one of the four partners is happy.

What was your main goal at the time you started in practice? Did you have one? Has it changed? In what way? What's your main goal today? Do you have one now? If so, is it *specific*? Is it *realistic*? Is it *flexible*? Does it have a *due date* attached? If your goal can't match all four of these criteria, you probably don't have a goal. You certainly don't have a workable goal. At best, you have a wish. And (sorry, Disney fans), "wishing" does *not* "make it so."

If your goal isn't specific, flexible, realistic and due-dated, restructure it — on paper, in writing. Be sure it measures up. If you have a goal but you don't like it, it's not working for you, or it worries you because you know you're not going to reach it, adjust it. It's flexible, remember?

Once you settle on a goal that makes sense, go get it! Brainwash yourself with your goal. Wake yourself up with it. Put yourself to sleep with it. Pace your exercise routine to it. Recite it to yourself as you walk or stand in line at the bank or wait for traffic lights. If someone woke you at 3 a.m. and asked you your goal, you should be able to rattle it off without hesitating.

Recite it to yourself in the present tense, as if you have already achieved it e.g., "I feel physically fit and mentally alert and I am enjoying all the benefits of weighing 168 pounds again." Envision yourself slim and trim. In preparation for board exams, your thought process might be something more along the lines of, "I am enjoying all the psychological and financial benefits of being board-certified," and envisioning your specialization certificate in your hands or framed and hanging on your office wall.

In your mind, picture yourself having already achieved your goal whenever you can. See every detail of this achievement in your mental image. Go over and over it until you can literally turn it on at will. Use every occasion (especially as you fall asleep and when you first awake) to reinforce your image.

If your goal, for instance, is to own an ocean-front estate ("I am enjoying living in the ocean-front home of my dreams that I love and can easily afford"), get a hold of some exclusive real estate photo ads (even copies of actual realtor listings in your dream location area) and study them. Imagine living in each. Find and cut out pictures of ocean-front estates to tack or tape up on your wall, mirror, closet door or refrigerator; put one behind your sun visor; put one in your wallet. One doctor has a large office bulletin board devoted to focusing on prospective dream houses and has her staff contributing photos and ads they run across (with a dinner-for-two limo trip for whomever brings in one that she ends up choosing). Repeated self-talk and repeated viewing of representations of your goal will strengthen and reinforce your commitment to achieve it.

Because you become what you think about.

Discovery: A Process Not Limited To Lawyers, Chemists, or 3-Year-Olds

Two of the most telling questions you can ask yourself (and those who work with you) is "What sport most closely resembles your (our) practice?" and "Why?" You're guaranteed to find the answers to these questions fascinating and, depending on how open-minded you're willing to be, illuminating.

One client of management consultant Dru Scott (as depicted in his video, *Transactional Analysis*, produced by McGraw-Hill) in response to these "What sport?" and "Why?" questions, said: "roller derby...because all we ever do is run around in circles, bash each other in the teeth, and put on a show for the public, but we never go anywhere."

And you can imagine the startled looks at one hospital's top management group meeting when one of the vice presidents, answering the same two questions, said: "sumo wrestling...because half our people struggle and push to move in one direction and the other half struggles and pushes to move in the opposite direction. We go a few steps forward, then a few steps backward, and the end result is no movement at all."

A talented young doctor who decided to relocate after having just completed his first year with an old, established group practice reported the group was "a marathon, because everyone is running on their own, at their own pace, for what seems like endless distances...we are all constantly tired and undernourished. And there's absolutely no teamwork."

This last example is not to suggest that if the "rookie" doctor's assessment of his group practice as a "marathon" had been made known to the practice's senior partners earlier in the year, they might have been able to secure the long-term contract they desired for him. Obviously, knowing what's wrong and doing something about it are two different things. But had someone asked the new doctor (or the senior partners) a simple "what sport is your practice" type of question even a couple of times during the year, odds are that appropriate adjustments might have been made. The loss of a potentially strong addition to the practice and the full year's investment in training and practice orientation could have been spared.

Thoughtful, simple, and often abstract questions can generate a flood of meaningful responses. They can prompt you to pause and reflect, reevaluate, reenergize, revitalize and reconstruct the direction in which your practice has been heading.

Evaluation: Weighing The Gray Matter

Whom do you presently rely on for advice? Include family, friends, associates and professional advisors (lawyers, accountants, practice and business consultants) in your thinking. What kinds of advice do they give you? At what point in the spectrum of problem development do you contact them? How frequently do you contact them?

The following exercise has four questions for you to respond to with a rating of 1-10 (1 = minimum; 10 = maximum), followed by some related questions to think about and some space for making notes.

ADVISORS

1. How satisfied are you with each advisor? _____
Who among your present advisors should you be looking to solidify relationships with even more? Who should you be looking to add or replace? What specific qualities will you seek in a new or replacement advisor? What deadline will you set for finding a new or replacement advisor? How much time and effort will you invest in "training" a new or replacement advisor? How much are you willing to pay a (professional) new or replacement advisor? Over what specific time period? To accomplish what specific tasks or contribute to what specific thinking?

_____

_____

_____

_____

_____

_____

_____

_____
_____
_____
_____
_____
_____
_____
_____
_____
_____
_____
_____

NUMBERS

2. How satisfied are you with your current revenues and Patient flow? _____

How far away are you from what the numbers should realistically be? What could they be ideally? What will it take to get there? What's standing in your way? How can you move, remove, or maneuver around the obstacles? How much time, energy and money are you willing to spend to get where you want to go? What do you *imagine* might be the first step you can take (to start improving your Patient and dollar flow numbers) this very minute, even before you start reading the next page?

_____
_____
_____
_____
_____
_____
_____
_____

_____

_____

_____

_____

_____

_____

_____

_____

_____

_____

_____

_____

IMAGE

3. How satisfied are you with your present image? _____
What do you think your image is? How different is your image from your reputation? What do you think your reputation is? When was the last time you checked with others about your image and reputation? Who did you check with? What exactly did you ask? Was your question a "loaded" one (like, "Would you agree that...?" or "Wouldn't you agree that...?")? Did you react or respond to the answers that were offered? How soon can you start to check your image again by asking more probing and more objective questions, and by being more receptive, less reactive, to answers you may not want to hear?

_____

_____

_____

_____

_____

_____

_____

_____

_____

_____

_____

_____

_____

_____

_____

_____

_____

_____

_____

_____

PERSONAL

4. How satisfied are you with your personal life right now? _____
Does your husband, wife or lover know exactly how you feel? Does this person genuinely understand? If you're holding back from him or her, are you automatically choosing to self-destruct by not sharing your life's most important feelings with your life's most important support system? How might you be choosing to do that? How can you reverse that attitude? What's the risk involved?

Given that a realistic fear is having a gun pointed at you, and that almost everything else is unrealistic because it's not here right now, how realistic is the risk involved? What will it take to get started with sharing your feelings, to not be so afraid of letting go? Are you making excuses? Are you, by keeping it all inside, choosing extinction?

Do the parents and children in your life really know what you're trying to do for yourself? Do they really know what you're trying to do for them? Have you clearly explained and carefully listened and thoroughly answered their questions? Are you making realistic judgements about how much they're capable of knowing, or need to know, or about how much they can or would be willing to contribute to help you be more satisfied? What would you want or expect from you if you were in their shoes right now?

What do you really know about how satisfied your husband, wife, lover, parents, and/or children are with their personal lives right now? What do you imagine they would want or expect from themselves if they were in your shoes right now?

_____

_____

_____

_____

_____

_____

_____

_____

_____

_____

_____

_____

_____

_____

_____

_____

_____

_____

_____

_____

What do the four rating numbers you wrote down as answers to the four questions suggest to you right now? What do the notes you jotted down suggest? If you didn't write anything, what do the blank lines suggest to you?

Describe the kinds of changes these rankings prompt you to think about. Write them down. Now. Then sleep on them. Then do them. If you think it's too hard to overcome the roadblocks, remember that *that's* a choice. You can choose for it to be easy. Anything less is an admission that circumstances, or other people, are reaching inside your head to "push your buttons" and control your brain. And, of course, only you can do that.

A View Through The Scope

In addition to choosing for changes to be easy, you can also choose for them to be fun and challenging. Take on one at a time. Start with the easiest to implement, then see it all the way through to completion before beginning with change number two. The reward for your focused attention will be positive feelings of accomplishment and enjoyment about your newfound sense of control and personal leadership.

Changes that you initiate can be sources of enormous energy, power, and excitement, vs. changes that are done *to* you, which to some, can seem (literally) life-threatening. Think about how resistant you feel when a hospital, insurance company, government agency, or other group you're subject to or affiliated with dictates a procedural change that you're obliged to follow. This thought is especially important to hold in your consciousness when you start making, or even suggesting, changes that will affect your staff. Don't not make the changes. But do be aware of the impact on people's psyches and sensitivities. Deal with them as you would want outside forces to deal with you.

By encouraging staff members to conceive and execute their own changes, you can expect them to feel more motivated and less threatened. Remember, the tasks you delegate and those you encourage others to invent, initiate, and pursue, don't have to be done exactly the way you would do them as long as the desired results are achieved in a safe and reasonable manner.

Compulsiveness breeds ineffective delegation ("Why did he ask me to do this job and then go ahead and do it himself?") and, often, behavioral backlash from support staff ("Next time he asks for something, I know he's going to end up doing it himself, so why should I even bother to try?"). The best way for you to let go of the fears you have for delegating decision-making responsibilities to your staff is to ask yourself: what's the worst that could happen? If your answer doesn't include some form of all-encompassing disaster, it's probably a safe bet that you can *let go* of your fears and distrust. And if the worst that can happen is, in fact, an event of major consequence, perhaps the function involved is not one that should be considered for delegation. Or perhaps it needs to be delegated "under observation," as a "monitoring arrangement," or on a trial or probationary basis.

If, on the other hand, you choose to disregard totally these considerations, you may want to take a moment to distance yourself from your interpersonal involvements with staff members long enough to objectively reassess the caliber of the people you have hired. If you're convinced that those who work for you are competent and worthwhile, and you *still* have problems delegating — with "letting go" — then it's time to explore your *own* ability to trust others. If you hit a dead end with this thinking, perhaps you should seek some professional guidance for ways to bolster this important shortcoming. If you honestly believe you have people working for you who cannot be trusted to take on additional responsibility, don't waste time keeping him/her/them past tomorrow — and exercise much greater care in recruiting any replacements.

Since delegation fears are primarily ego-related, it's generally better to view the act of delegating as simply affording someone else the chance to learn how to do a responsible task that will spare you the effort of doing it and provide that person with a new opportunity to grow. To the outside world, by the way, you also tend to appear more professional when those around you are handling responsibilities that are clearly professional.

Ticktock, Ticktock...

As most doctors know from the unhappy thoughts that accompany the examination of legal bills, "delay" is the lawyer's modus operandi. (The longer the delays, the higher the lawyer's fees.) Government, and most service industries would have us believe that delays are normal, to be expected, and pardonable. The tendency most physicians have to delay, postpone, avoid, or completely gloss over personal growth and relationship problems could easily and mistakenly influence you to believe that: A) It's okay to not deal with the reality of personal tangles;

and B) Professional/practice/business issues and/or personal development opportunities should also be put off whenever possible.

Nothing could be farther from the truth. In both business and personal growth pursuits, act like you're in the E.R. We know many successful clinicians, business leaders, and psychotherapists who all share the exact same motto: *Some Action Is Better Than No Action.* "No Action" is more than just standing still. It literally is an investment in maintaining the status quo. It's the process of intentionally shriveling up. It's the process of going nowhere. If you never let go, nothing will grow.

What differences are there in Patient perceptions about you, your practice, your skills, reputation and personality vs. Staff perceptions? Vs. community perceptions? How does your family view you? When was the last time you asked family members for some honest feedback and then actually took it in and processed it, receptively and appreciatively? When was the last time you specifically asked a few Patients and Staff people *how* you "come across" to others?

One doctor, for example, was told by a Patient that she had a handshake "like a wet fish." Rather than act insulted, she asked the Patient to teach her how he would like to have her shake his hand. He did. She reports that more people now seem to treat her "more forthrightly and more respectfully than in my fish-shake days."

Satisfaction: The Tuba and The Lard

One revealing evaluation device is to ask your Patients or Staff, "What kind of animal (or musical instrument or food or drink or movie title) would you associate with me, and why?" Whatever the answers, even if they're: "Snake, because you're slithery and sleazy," "Tuba, because you're always blowing hot air," "Lard, because you're totally fat and greasy," "Kamikaze, because you're killing yourself with drinking, smoking, junk food and temper tantrums," or "Gone With The Wind, because you disappear whenever a business question comes up," be prepared to take it on the chin, gracefully, good-naturedly, humbly (yes, humbly), quietly, and, of course, appreciatively. Remember, it's harder, riskier, and more psychologically threatening for most people to provide honest feedback than it is to take it!

Think about the feedback you get. Don't discuss it with the Patient or staff member unless it's to ask for clarification or an example. Certainly don't argue about it. Just think about it. Surprise, spontaneous responses such as these can be great teachers!

Do A Diagnostic Workup

If you don't know enough about what's going on in the various areas of your life, enough to be able to jot down quick, meaningful summary notes on each, then you don't know enough to prompt meaningful increases in Patient and income flow. So take some steps on your own behalf before you start seeking to influence others. It's time to learn more about your self.

Take your professional temperature. You need to start tomorrow morning and spend the next full week being a detective. Quietly look and listen everywhere for clues. Gather enough evidence in every category to support your summary notes (the ones you've been recording in your "History Notebook" that you started earlier in this book, but that it's not too late to start now if you've just been caught in the act of avoidance).

What should you jot down? Here's an example: What are the kinds of circumstances that tend to set you up to choose anger as a response? What specific statements, thoughts and situations tend to set you up to be consistently happy and pleasant and productive all day long? Be especially honest with yourself on these points. Your answers will give you important clues.

As stated previously, getting your answers and other thoughts written down on paper takes them, and all the accompanying clutter, out of your head. This seems to have the effect of leaving more room in your brain for it to focus on more immediate issues, like your health, your family, and your Patients.

Take your professional pulse. You need to start doing this right now. Put the book down and take a quick five minute walk through your office. A real walk is best, but even closing your eyes and imagining it will do for the moment. Pretend you're seeing your office for the very first time. What does your mind take in when you "step back" like this mentally? What do the images communicate? Is the "pulse" steady or erratic? For instance, are the plants in your office reception area being properly cared for? (Live plants, by the way, communicate aliveness; dump the fake ones immediately!) Are the reading materials current and in good condition? Last week's beat up newspaper and six month-old, torn-up magazines don't do much to create the impression of you as a doctor who's "up on all the latest" and who's neat, clean, and organized.

If you offer office visitors music, a TV, or a fish tank, be 100% sure they're in A-1 condition every day, all day long. Be sure someone on the staff takes responsibility for this at all times. Imagine the impression (and stress) people get from static-filled speakers, a fuzzy television screen, or even worse, dead fish floating in the tank. One doctor discovered the state of his office this way:

> As I laid back on the same examination table I hover over each day, to catch a quick nap while my staff had gone to lunch, I was horrified to see smudged spotlights, a torn drapery valance, a cobweb in the ceiling corner, and a large, dead cockroach laying spread-eagle inside the fluorescent light cover. Now I look up automatically as I come in each morning. I wouldn't want a Patient to associate me with dirt, bugs, and torn fabric.

A dirty reception area communicates a dirty doctor. Worn out furnishings communicate a worn out doctor. Gossipy front desk personnel communicate a doctor with no regard for privacy. I'm reminded of an orthodontist's sign I saw recently that had crooked lettering and broken support posts (the wood appeared to be rotted) that had been sistered together with some mismatched two by fours. Can you imagine Patient's impressions of what this dentist might do to straighten out their teeth?

Check your professional blood pressure. Put the sleeve around your practice and pump up the little rubber squeeze ball. Watch the dial. Better yet, put a handkerchief over your home phone mouthpiece one morning and give your office a call. Some doctors make a practice of doing this on a regular basis. Ask for information about the doctor and see what you hear about yourself. Ask for when the next available appointment. Ask for rates and information about how insurance and Medicare paperwork is handled.

Bite your tongue if need be, but don't reveal who you are. Listen instead. Listen between the lines. Listen carefully for how the information is presented. Then, after you hang up, take some time to process what was communicated, and how it was done. Think for awhile about the impressions someone made on you about your self and your own practice.

The Most Effective "Telemarketing" is Quiet, Unscripted, and Personal

An occasional voice-disguised night call to your answering service can be illuminating too, as this doctor found out:

> I phoned my office one Sunday afternoon to see how the

calls were being handled. There was laughter in my ear the minute I heard a connection. When the operator finally answered, she couldn't pronounce the name of my practice. When I told her the call was an emergency, she was so preoccupied with continuing her laughing (along with two or three others I could hear in the background) that she completely missed what I said, and actually put me on hold for nearly two minutes. Needless to say, I had alternative phone answering arrangements in place by Monday morning.

You must know exactly how your front desk phone is being answered, word for word. After you check it out, ask others what they hear when they call. You must be certain that the person answering your phones is consistently projecting the right personality and attitude, as well as a sense of urgency, empathy, and professionalism to fit the image you want others to have of you with every single call.

Prospective Patients' first impressions of you are based 100% on how your phone is answered. A telephone personality that registers a friendly, positive, understanding attitude and an appropriate sense of confidence and urgency is at least as important as the words that are said. [Note to the reader: Please do the medical profession a favor by photocopying this paragraph and sending it to your colleagues who insist on acting like a telecommunications complex by relying on voice mail instead of real, live people to answer their phones. Not only do other professionals dislike voice mail systems, Patients hate them! For an illustration of a ludicrous script one doctor is actually using, see the "Voicemailmonster" on page 135.]

Existing and past Patients look for recognition and reassurance when they call. This shouldn't surprise you. Don't you also seek recognition and reassurance when you are a repeat customer? Doesn't a genuinely warm greeting (especially by name) at the door of your favorite restaurant make you feel good? This is not to suggest that you're running a restaurant. But Patients rightfully believe they're entitled to expect these same accommodating, warm, restaurateur-type qualities from you and your staff. In fact, your role as healer, in your Patients' eyes, makes it your *job* to be nurturing and to treat your "customers" with extra attentiveness.

Consider that when you call a place of business, the person answering the phone actually *becomes* the business in your mind. In the same fashion, *your receptionist is your practice* to every caller. In fact, many callers won't mentally separate you from your receptionist. When callers phone a doctor's office and get an untrained, matter-of-fact-sounding bimbo or bozo who is preoccupied with front desk chit-chat, a piece of bubble gum, or an on-hold personal call, disrespect and inattentiveness are immediately associated with the doctor.

Altogether too many medical receptionists act like they've never experienced feelings of embarrassment themselves when calling a doctor. "And what seems to be the trouble?" comes the typical receptionist response, not much unlike the kind of question you might expect from a greasy-spoon waitress when you ask to send back your profusely bleeding hamburger.

Remember that the Patient is being asked rather bluntly what they may consider to be a highly personal question. Even worse, it's coming from a mysterious receptionist-type person who answered the phone, someone who is not the doctor, who the caller doesn't even know, much less trust. And let's say that the caller is trying to schedule an examination for a prostate condition that he is so afraid or embarrassed to deal with that he had to raise major muster even to pick up the phone in the first place, let alone discuss the details with a total stranger. Even worse, the receptionist might just turn out to be his neighbor's daughter!

How much more reassuring a response such as this would be: "My name is Copa Setic. I am Dr. Softouch's receptionist. He's asked me to take this call for him and write down what you tell me so he can review your concerns and questions on his very next break between appointments. Let's start with your name and phone number, and then we'll see if I can help you describe the problem you would like me to tell the doctor about." Sure, it takes more time and energy to say something like this. Good, productive, sensitive communications always require more work and take longer than poor, nonproductive, insensitive communications. But the former will never cost you a single Patient. The latter will cost you many. And anything that costs you "many" also costs you *money*, guaranteed.

Speaking of costs, be assured that no practice in the world has ever prospered simply by cutting corners. You don't make money by conserving on electricity, cutting back on advertising and staff training expenses, or by limiting staff phone calls, break time, or free coffee. You make money by making money. Assuming you don't function out of a nonprofit entity that can look to fund-raising donations as a source of income, there are only two ways to increase revenues: 1) Increase fees, which of course has legal and ethical ceilings; and 2) Increase patient flow, which is limited only by your clinical skills, your ability to work hard and delegate effectively, and by the consistency with which you devote yourself to building and strengthening Patient relationships.

Take the story of one large (but shrinking) group practice that continually refuses to capitalize on its own marketing successes. The practice director ignores Patient flow increases stimulated by the combined promotional and public relations efforts of a savvy staff and talented outside professionals. And he is rewarded not for actually generating income based on dollars earned, but based solely on his ability to cut practice expenses. For this, the practice partners compensate the practice director with $200,000 a year (on top of his annual practice income which exceeds $400,000!).

Not only is $200,000 a scandalous amount of money for doing nothing (which is, in essence, what this person does), it certainly doesn't say much for the mentality of the misguided partners who vote annually on the directorship fee as a reward for reducing expenses. "It's a government mentality," laments the practice's frustrated business manager.

"The real issue in this situation is obviously one of greed," observes a well-informed executive with the group's affiliate hospital. "The partners' lack of business sense sets up a fantasy that suggests to them that they could each take home more money if they didn't have to pay their marketing people (who I happen to know are getting good, dollar-productive results) and that they could each take home more money if they didn't have to pay the media and production expenses that I understand are just a tiny fraction of the new patient revenues being generated," she says. "The ludicrousness of their shortsightedness is matched only by their belief that the $200,000 is well spent. They would do better to each take home chunks of the $200,000 and do away with the director's fee."

Even though the practice had not been experiencing any kind of financial crunch, and even though expenses had been conscientiously kept under control by responsible and dedicated employees and by value-conscious outside service providers, the doctor/practice director was so anxious to justify his worth to his partners that he began to cut expenses with reckless abandon.

Three months prior to his contract renewal vote, he eliminated the $150,000 advertising and public relations programs that were bringing in $2,500,000 worth of new and referral Patient revenues.

Four months prior to his contract renewal vote, he eliminated backup switchboard employees in favor of a less expensive, but highly impersonal and user-complicated voice mail system.

He eliminated the last quarter of a quarterly Patient newsletter series, without regard for it's pointed promotion in the first, second, and third quarter issues of "The Special Year-End Edition" that would feature "Important New Information For Every Family."

He eliminated employee bonuses, two paid holidays, and pension fund contributions for six months prior to his contract renewal vote, sending employee morale plummeting and the best employees in search of new employment.

To what avail, all of this chopping and hacking away? Frugality? Thriftiness? Economic belt tightening? Rehearsing to run for political office? Or just plain greed? The result of this cost-cutting was that the practice began functioning like a stereotypical nonproductive, inefficient, lethargic government agency. None of the doctors could figure out why Patient and dollar volume were fading away. They blamed it on the economy. But at least they succeeded in reducing expenses, they thought.

At some point in the not-too-distant future, the partners will still be paying the practice director $200,000 a year, and wondering what went wrong when they're forced to file for bankruptcy.

Feel For Lumps

Step back from your practice and assess your aches and pains. Be honest with yourself. You need to know clearly what the weakest, most vulnerable areas are. You can't improve a weakness you don't know exists, or are afraid to admit to. Seek out the "lumps" objectively, scientifically, and categorically.

As you assess and diagnose, don't choose to get caught up in emotional issues and reactions. If you don't react (vs. respond), it's impossible to overreact, and this applies to every situation in life. If you don't *over*react, you probably won't get yourself in trouble with other people. You will most certainly live longer.

Now, you're probably saying to yourself that all this is easy to say, but how do you consciously *not* react? The following dialogue from a scrub-up session will give you a hint:

Nurse: Say, Doc, do you mind if I tell you something I've noticed about you?
Doctor: (kidding) Shouldn't we wait until after we've done this

gallbladder?

Nurse: (smiling) No, I mean besides that I think you're cute. I've wondered whether you realize that from the time you ask for the scalpel (sometimes you wait until the clamps) until the time you close up, your teeth are clenched. And — I know this sounds ridiculous — you look like you're not breathing. (Both turn serious as they face each other.) Anyway, I felt worried about that and thought I should mention it. I hope you don't believe in shooting the messenger or anything. I mean, I'm only mentioning this because of the yoga course I'm taking.

Doctor: Thanks. I guess maybe I have been holding my breath a lot lately. It's been hard keeping my mind off my son. I keep thinking that his getting busted for drugs might not have happened if I had done something differently, like spend more time with him, you know?

Nurse: I know, Doc, but it's not too late to start. Besides, you can't change what's already happened. Anyway, I thought you should know it shows.

Doctor: I really do appreciate you bringing it to my attention. Is there anything else I should know from that yoga course of yours?

(both smiling again)

Nurse: Actually, you just need to remember to ask yourself one question every time we go into the operating room...

IV

ARE YOU BREATHING?

If you can breathe more deeply every day, you will think more clearly, perform more confidently, feel more relaxed, and be more productive more often. You will be healthier, happier, and have greater control of your mind, body, emotions and circumstances.

Try This

1. Sitting or standing, feet flat on the floor and hands resting comfortably at your sides, close your mouth and take a slow deep breath in through your nose.

2. Instead of directing the air that you take in, as you normally would, to the top part of your lungs, fill the bottom part of your lungs so that your stomach sticks out instead of your chest.

3. Now shift the air up to the top part of your lungs so that your stomach is in and your chest is out. Hold it there a few seconds, then loosen your jaw and exhale through your mouth in a slow, steady stream — you need to be able to hear yourself do this.

4. When you think you've exhaled all the air, don't believe yourself; there's more inside. Give an extra little push or two to exhale. It's this extra push that does the trick, that makes this exercise work so well. Then close your mouth and repeat the process until you're able to hear yourself exhale smoothly and evenly, with no little hitches in air flow.

Go slowly at first, the same way you would begin any new exercise. If you experience slight dizziness or excessive coughing, don't be alarmed; simply return to your "normal" way of breathing. But you should realize that these "signals" indicate you could probably benefit even more than most people by making additional attempts to master this mother of all methods of self-management.

If you're a smoker, you may actually see smoke come out when you exhale deeply. Realize that your "normal" breathing does absolutely nothing for that cloud you've been carrying around in the bottom of your lungs. Take the time to appreciate how good it feels to clear your lungs out.

It's normal that a first attempt at this process might be somewhat awkward, jerky, and/or exaggerated. With practice, you'll be able to take these deep breaths as most athletes and performers do — "on the spot" and "routinely" in stressful situations, without having to exaggerate each step, as you may be doing now. Odds are, in fact, that no one will ever notice. If someone should happen to see you and ask what you're doing, "I'm breathing" is always a great answer that's hard for anyone to find fault with.

You will also gain increased breathing control if you focus your mind on silently repeating to yourself: "Energy in, energy in, energy in..." with each inhalation, and "Tension out, tension out, tension out..." with each exhalation. It's worth pointing out here that a great many doctors who use and teach deep breathing to Patients report that Patients who concentrate on their ailments (by repeating to themselves, for example, "Energy into my shoulder, tension out of my shoulder" or "Energy into my colon, tension out of my colon") as they do the breathing, actually heal quicker than those who try to mentally "tune out" or "push away" pain and discomfort.

What's so magical about all this breathing? Nothing that ancient yogis didn't know, or Lamaze birthing instructors, or mountain climbers, or baseball pitchers as they wind up, or football linemen as they wait for the snap, or actors as they prepare to come on stage. The fact is, it works. Every deep breath increases blood and oxygen circulation, which relaxes your muscles, makes your brain more alert, and soothes your neurological system. Every deep breath you take increases your personal productivity by increasing your mental focus on "here and now," on the present moment, on what's right in front of you. After all, along with your pulse and heartbeat, your breathing is the most immediate "here and now" thing happening in your life.

Remember, if you can train yourself to take deep breaths in response to stressful situations, you will be responding instead of reacting. When you can prevent yourself from reacting, you automatically eliminate the risk of overreacting.

Some of the best times and places to practice breathing are in the car (to be more in tune with the road and traffic), before opening a door (to be better prepared for whatever or whomever might be on the other side), before dictating diagnostic or treatment notes (to help ensure that you are communicating accurately), before answering the phone or checking phone messages (to be better prepared for whatever you may hear), before — and while — dealing with an upset, angry, or irate partner, associate, staff person, Patient or Patient family member (to stay in better control of yourself), at bedtime (to help clear your mind and get to sleep quicker), when you wake up (to help you move and think more alertly, more quickly), during time spent with children (to more quickly shed the rigidity of being grown up and more readily communicate at an acceptable level; in case you've forgotten about adult rigidity getting in the way of child relations, see the movie *Hook* starring Robin Williams), and during lovemaking, especially breathing in tandem with your partner (to help you feel more and think less).

Many surgical team members and trauma specialists have also found success with the use of deep breathing just before entering the O.R. (or E.R.), and during surgical procedures as well.

Many trauma victims reportedly have saved themselves from going into shock by remembering or being prodded to take deep breaths. A 19-year-old woman who was thrown over 30 feet from her car on crash impact, was told by three different doctors after she had completely recovered that she would have died from shock had she not focused every ounce of energy on taking deep breaths. A nearly identical story came from a 47-year-old man who was pinned inside an overturned car for three hours and who was coaxed and coached into deep breathing by an otherwise helpless passerby who used the technique for calming down the elementary school children she taught. A back-on-the-job "breathing and stress management-trained" undercover state trooper was shot twice and left for dead in an alleyway drug bust attempt; deep breathing reportedly saved him...and on and on.

Deep breathing is a tool to help you do more with what you've got. A page on my calendar says: "*Success is the maximum utilization of the ability that you have* — Zig Ziglar." Remind yourself that no matter what your age or level of health or fitness, your mind and your body are capable of accomplishing a great deal more than you probably believe is possible.

This is not to suggest you will suddenly become a mystic or psychic or that you leap out of your daily home routine or work setting to compete in the Olympics. But there is a message here that once you have mastered this deep breathing technique and can "plug it in" to stressful moments, once you begin to build deep breathing into your day-to-day lifestyle activities, you will begin to help yourself perform better at every level of what you do in life for work and play and even sleep. The bottom line is that if this works for you as first aid, it works even better as a permanent life-enhancer and problem-preventer.

The best way to remind yourself to breathe deep is to teach others. When you show Patients how to use this technique (not just tell them, but actually demonstrate the technique and coach them through two or three breaths), you are making your job easier. A Patient who understands and uses deep breathing will be more relaxed during examination and treatment. By teaching Patients, you are giving them something specific they can use to help themselves get better quicker. You are also giving them a valuable lifelong gift of self-control and self-reliance. They will think and speak of you as doctor *and* mentor. They will think of you more often, quite possibly, with every conscious deep breath. (No amount of advertising can accomplish that!)

Encourage Patients, family members, and associates you teach, to in turn, teach others. You will be cited as the source. Not only will you be Johnny Appleseeding your community, you will be generating and realizing new referrals to your practice without spending a penny on marketing! Try it consistently, every day, for several weeks. Watch what happens. You have nothing to lose — except stress.

When family members and work associates understand and practice deep breathing, positive changes and attitudes abound. Everyone can take shared responsibility for reminding one another when someone appears to be out of sorts to simply ask the innocent, nonthreatening, caring question, "Are You Breathing?"

Triage Yourself

When it's time for first aid, do it. But, no more than you would hold gauze pads on a gaping wound longer than it takes to get it cleaned out and sutured, be realistic enough to appreciate that temporary relief for the business part of your practice is only temporary.

When an oral surgeon pulls a tooth, a new one grows in to replace it, or an implant or false tooth is used to replace it, or the Patient learns to live without it. In business, even permanent relief is temporary. When a "tooth is pulled" (such as firing your front desk person), every other "tooth" (or staff person) can rot or fall out within a matter of days, even hours!

On the flip side, keep in mind that *without* the "extraction" in the first place, the "bad tooth" will definitely get worse, and will eventually rot all the others anyway. So, whatever your decision, make it promptly (and generously, so it doesn't come back to haunt you) and don't delay taking action, medical-emergency style. In business, the process is called "cutting your losses."

Next you need to inform all those who are directly affected by your decision: A) what your decision is and why, and B) that you need their confidence, trust, and help to get through the upset period. Have this meeting *immediately* (the same day). Be *careful* with the tone of voice and the words you use to explain things (keep it brief and matter-of-fact). Make it a point to conduct the meeting *personally* (vs. by representative or written notice), even if you must interrupt your Patient schedule.

Specifically, ask your people to rise to the occasion, to pitch in and cover the extra work load, until the "extracted tooth" can be replaced. Tell them you'll reward them accordingly. Then make sure you *do it.* [It's worth keeping in mind here that free lunches during this period often can go a long way toward motivating staff teamwork and offsetting the need to provide financial incentives.]

By following through with rewards for employees who rally to your call, you are reassuring them of your loyalty to them, and of your own sense of integrity. You must also, however, be sure to "follow through" the entire incident by exercising greater care than in the past with your personnel recruitment, evaluation, and selection efforts — and especially with your arrangements for proper training. Putting more time, attention, and energy into these beginning processes may be the *only* way to prevent future staff uproars.

Of course, soliciting and considering the impressions of others is important, but we always recommend that the doctor or, in the case of a larger practice, the medical director, make *all* final hiring decisions. It's fine to weigh the input and opinions of others, but in the end *every* employee is your personal representative to the outside world.

To the shock and dismay of many doctors who learn the hard way, it is *not* true that employees are the office or practice manager's personal representatives to the outside world. You need to know that your staff people are loyal to *you.* Too many practices are undermined by over-zealous or manipulative administrators. And you know where that road leads that's "paved with good intentions."

Disgruntled employees who have been removed from key positions often have created havoc with Patient flow by vindictively spreading negative rumors. Some have helped to create tomorrow's headlines by making anonymous, unfounded complaints to local news reporters. Worst of all, a few have seen fit to ignite Gestapo-style inquiries by taking their phoney complaints to peer review organizations and state medical boards of examiners, who tend to condemn first and investigate second. There are enough SMBE and PRO horror stories to fill the rest of this book, but you undoubtedly know your own.

V

QUIET MEDICAL MARKETING

"Waiting" For Patients

Altogether too many doctors still have the unrealistic notion that they need only "hang out a shingle" to attract Patients. This kind of fantasizing tends to be most prevalent with brand new, fresh-out-of-med-school graduates who are setting up private practices, but the sense of naivete it represents is also often found among older, more established doctors and many mature group practices.

Maybe you don't need an MBA after your doctor credentials, but being a nonmarketing/nonmanagement-savvy professional doesn't work anymore. While you're waiting for a Patient to decide to come to you, he or she is being bombarded by messages from more aggressive competitors. This is being accomplished through the persuasive use of seminar talks, health fairs and shows, brochures, direct mail, radio and cable television commercials, newspaper and magazine ads, custom-printed promotional items, telemarketing presentations, and even billboards. There's even a doctor who advertises, Lord save us, on matchbook covers.

To ignore the impact of all this, to not be actively engaged in marketing your practice is, as the old country singer Tennessee Ernie Ford once described "trouble," like being "a long-tailed cat in a room full of rockin' chairs." Low profile advertising is fine, but such independence can only be worthwhile when you compensate with personalized attention to Patients and staff, with total immersion in community activities (supported by ongoing public relations efforts), and when your overall approach is a realistic one.

Think of it this way: *Not marketing your practice is like not brushing your teeth.* If you ignore marketing your practice, it will rot and fall apart.

To be a successful, marketing-savvy professional, you need to realize that effective marketing, marketing that delivers true dollar value, is not just the implementation of some newspaper ads and the printing of a brochure. Unless the message you put out is reinforced at every level of your practice, every minute of every day, you're not doing marketing; you're simply running some newspaper ads and printing a brochure.

Often this little promotional "dabbling" works better than nothing, but by itself, it will never do you justice. Effective marketing means representing the uniqueness *and* the totality of your practice by every legal, cost-effective way imaginable to your target Patient or Patient group, throughout the year, and in a constant and consistent manner.

Consistency means every level: *visually*, in the colors and typefaces that represent your logo, your office decor and signs, all of your printed materials (including letterhead, envelopes, invoices, folders, brochures, newsletters, ads, business and appointment cards, referral and announcement cards, magnets and other promotional items, etc.), even the colors and styles of staff lab jackets and name badges; *audibly*, in the form, content, market reach, and message frequency of what you say one-on-one with Patients, staff, and associates, as well as with audiences of any size, and especially with broadcast commercials and interviews.

And in terms of news releases, one release a year will not get published as readily as one a month because even the media seek consistency before giving recognition in the form of printing your information.

Some might argue that seasonality is a factor for some specialties. More bone injuries in the summer and winter doesn't mean orthopods can avoid showing their faces in the spring and fall. People unconsciously shop for doctors 365 days a year. It's often a topic of conversation at private family gatherings, in between toasts and desserts. More than one Thanksgiving or Christmas dinner, wedding, birthday, anniversary, and bar mitzvah have witnessed lengthy discussions on some doctor's bedside manners.

For the sake of an image anchored in consistency, it's better to start an ambitious program of monthly seminars with only five or six people at each, than to conduct one big bash that attracts 25 or 30 people. Don't think that talking with small gatherings is a costly waste of your time. You're not Charlton Heston or Richard Burton. Your medical hour value is not the same as your speaking hour value (unless you're somehow scheduling talks during your normal doctoring times).

Whatever your marketing message, it must measure up to the guideline, "A.I.D.A.S.," which stands for:

Attention — does it attract the attention of the target group of prospective Patients and/or referring professionals you seek to reach?

Interest — does it create interest with your target group?

Desire — does it stimulate desire in a manner your target group will relate to?

Action — does it bring about action by providing a specific step to take, address to visit or write to, or phone number to call?

Satisfaction — does it cultivate satisfaction by ensuring prompt, thorough, comfortable and convenient Patient care?

Figure 5-1 illustrates a two-sided printed page that was used as a combination newspaper insert/flyer/handout/direct mail piece. The promotional piece's focus of rewarding people for participating in a community service program is what captured initial attention. The text copy and "Sponsor's Message" created interest. The list of prizes served to stimulate desire. The "How To Win, And Where To Take Your No-Longer Used Glasses" box, plus a "Drop Off Locations" listing and prominent appearances of the phone number were all ways to bring about action. And satisfaction is cultivated throughout with references to helping needy people and to having multiple chances to win prizes.

This program, in fact, went many miles beyond just being effective. It was a complete "win-win" situation for all involved. Donor businesses received positive public exposure (accompanying news releases featured them as "community good guys"). Eyeglass lens and frame donors profited personally by knowing that recycling could make it possible for needy people to benefit by their old, unused glasses, and that they would get numerous chances to win valuable prizes for donating the old glasses. Needy, underprivileged people who received the glasses would benefit with better vision, at no cost. And the doctor, who sought positive community image publicity, gained more stature and respect in the senior marketplace (the market his specialty caters to) than he could have attracted with a million dollar advertising campaign.

On top of it all, the doctor gave each participating business a personalized, engraved appreciation plaque (showing his own name as well, of course). Years later, most of these plaques still hang in storefronts and offices as permanent "silent salesmen."

When Shock Treatment Fails, Try A Lobotomy

Once, at a small social gathering, a friend approached me "in confidence" as he put it. Glancing around, he smiled nervously and whispered "Would

Figure 5-1 front

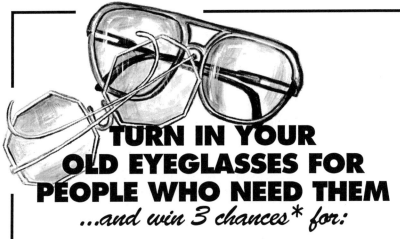

TURN IN YOUR OLD EYEGLASSES FOR PEOPLE WHO NEED THEM
...and win 3 chances* for:

*

Chances based on 1 entry coupon provided for each lens (sorry, no "contacts") and each frame contributed

Random drawing to be conducted Sunday, July 22, at 2:20 p.m. in the parking lot of the Americana Motel, 925 Rt. 166 (Rt. 9) Toms River

- A FREE WEEK'S STAY FOR YOUR NEXT FAMILY OR FRIENDS' VISIT (OR YOURSELF) AT THE NEWLY RENOVATED AMERICANA MOTEL
- A PAIR OF LOVEBIRDS, COMPLETE WITH DECORATIVE CAGE AND FULL SUPPLIES FROM FANCY SCHMANCY'S PET STORE
- A FULLY CATERED LUNCHEON FOR 6 DELIVERED TO YOUR FRONT DOOR FROM SMELLY BELLY EAT-IN DELI
- A COMPLETE OUTDOOR BARBECUE GRILL SET-UP FROM THE COMPLETE OUTDOOR BARBECUE SET-UP COMPANY
- YOUR CHOICE OF TAKE-OUT OR TABLE SERVICE DINNER FOR TWO FROM CHOP STIX CHINESE RESTAURANT
- QUALITY CLEANING OF ANY 3 WASHABLE ITEMS TOO LARGE FOR YOUR HOME WASHER AND DRYER. FROM DIRTY DUD'S COIN-OP AND COMMERCIAL LAUNDRY.
- A COMPLETE SELECTION OF TOP QUALITY COSMETICS FROM SLUG'S DRUGS.
- 3 DOZEN FREE GAME PLAYS FROM CARPEL TUNNEL ARCADE FAMILY AMUSEMENTS
- ...SEE REVERSE SIDE FOR MORE PRIZES AND DETAILS.

Have you ever thought about recycling those old eyeglasses you have stored away to help someone else who needs them but who can't afford to buy them?

Now's your chance to help us help the ongoing collection drives of Community Good Deed Clubs... to help some underprivileged, glasses-needy people... *and win a valuable prize for your thoughtfulness!*

PLEASE DON'T THROW THIS FLYER AWAY... See the reverse side for complete prize list, rules, drop-off locations, drawing information, etc.... **THEN PASS IT ALONG OR POST IT!**

ALL PRIZES DONATED AS A COMMUNITY SERVICE BY THE BUSINESSES AND INDIVIDUALS IDENTIFIED. PROGRAM EXCLUSIVELY SPONSORED AND PAID FOR AS A SERVICE TO THE COMMUNITY BY:

EYE, EYE, EYE, EYE HEALTH CENTER
With Experience, Skill and Technology: We Listen. We Care. We Help.
364-2020

Figure 5-1 back

Continued from opposite side...

MORE PRIZES...

- AN AUTHENTIC ANTIQUE TEDDY BEAR AND A BAGFUL OF "PENNY CANDY" FROM GRIN & BEAR IT GENERAL STORE
- A COMPLETE SUB SANDWICH PICNIC FOR 4 FROM THE SUB SANDWICH PICNIC FOR 4 STORE
- A FULL HAIRSTYLING TREATMENT FROM HAIR TODAY-GONE TOMORROW HAIR STYLISTS
- A QUALITY-GUARANTEED PRINTING OF 1,000 BUSINESS CARDS, OR 100 INVITATIONS FROM SMUDGE 'N SMEAR PRINTERS
- FREE BEND OVER BACKWARD EXERCISE TAPE BY DR. D. OUBLEJOINT FROM RACKEM N' CRACKEM CHIROPRACTIC CENTER
- A $100 SAVINGS BOND FROM LAST NATIONAL BANK
- A BRAND NEW $50 BILL FROM STRINGS ATTACHED ACCOUNTING AND TAX SERVICES
- APPRECIATION PLAQUES FOR "MOST LENSES" AND "OLDEST FRAMES" FROM "GOLD-STAR-FOR-YOUR-FOREHEAD" TROPHIES & PLAQUES
- *...AND THE LIST KEEPS GROWING. WATCH YOUR LOCAL NEWSPAPERS FOR UPCOMING NEWS STORIES ON ADDITIONAL PRIZES*

HOW TO WIN, AND WHERE TO TAKE YOUR NO-LONGER USED GLASSES...

1. Turn in your old eyeglass lenses (sorry, no contacts) and frames at any of the locations shown below.
2. You will receive one drawing coupon for each lens and one for each frame.
3. Fill out each coupon and deposit in the box provided.
4. Winners will be announced on July 22 (See box on reverse side of flyer) and notified by phone.

DROP OFF LOCATIONS...

- **EYE, EYE, EYE, EYE HEALTH CENTER**
One Professional Plaza
1200 Rt. 5
- **AMERICANA MOTEL**
Rt. 166
- **GRIN & BEAR IT GENERAL STORE**
515 Bay Avenue
- **SMELLY BELLY DELI**
Brick Blvd. and Cedar Bridge Ave.
- **THE COMPLETE OUTDOOR BARBECUE GRILL SETUP COMPANY**
Todd/Last National Bank Plaza •
1091 Rt. 9
- **HAIR TODAY-GONE TOMORROW HAIR STYLISTS**
Oakridge-Rt. 37

SPONSOR'S MESSAGE

As you may have heard, our staff has been caught up in the excitement of having recently introduced a brand new innovative technological method of removing cataracts with a "NO-STITCHES" surgery technique, which will be available in June.

DR. C. ROOKEDLOOKIN

We decided to see if we could transfer some of the energy and enthusiasm we have for this exciting new development and try to mobilize the faith we have in the people of this county by taking a more active leadership role in sponsoring the program described in this flyer.

The response from our community – both businesses and individuals – has been overwhelming.

Early indications are that we may be able to help as many as 10,000 eyeglass-needy, underprivileged people to see more clearly than they've been able to for years...in some cases, for their entire lives ... thanks to Community Good Deed Club efforts and yours!

On behalf of all those involved, I extend my sincerest appreciation for your generosity...and keep digging out those old, no-longer, used eyeglasses ...let's make everyone a winner!

C. Rookedlookin, M.D.

P.S. Additional prize donations will be gratefully appreciated and publicized.
Call 364-2020

ALL PRIZES DONATED AS A COMMUNITY SERVICE BY THE BUSINESSES AND INDIVIDUALS IDENTIFIED. PROGRAM EXCLUSIVELY SPONSORED AND PAID FOR AS A SERVICE TO THE COMMUNITY BY:

EYE, EYE, EYE, EYE HEALTH CENTER
With Experience, Skill and Technology: We Listen. We Care. We Help.
364-2020

you please stop in to visit my brother? He's a brand new doctor and he really doesn't know much about getting started. My family and I have tried everything we could think of to help him get off and running, but he's been so resistant. We've actually reached the point of trying to shock him into taking action, but all that does is make him, and all of us, frustrated and irritable." My friend went on, "We just don't know how to get the message through to him that he needs to take some steps on his own behalf to get his practice going. Just let me know what's involved. I'll pay for whatever he needs. Here's his name and address."

Little did my friend know that by all rights I should have submitted a bill for performing a business lobotomy — which is what it turned out was needed. When I arrived at the new doctor's address, I found him — only by trusting his brother's directions — in a small, hand-printed, cardboard sign-marked room at the end of the hall, behind a fly-by-night-looking real estate office.

He was sitting quietly behind an old, drab green, dented, metal Army surplus desk (in a matching chair) with a single rickety wooden chair (clearly a flea market bargain) propped next to his desk for visitors, and a flimsy folding examination table that seemed to float ominously in the middle of his otherwise vacant, bare-floored "office."

As I entered the office, he stood up from behind a two foot-high pile of magazines and grinned. "Hi!," he said. "My brother told me you were coming." I smiled back. We shook hands. He gestured to the magazines. "They're mostly free samples I'm considering for subscriptions...as soon as they're affordable," he added apologetically, pushing the stack aside. After mumbling another sentence or two, he fumbled awkwardly through a description of what he was capable of and what he wanted to achieve, which included an objective of having fifty patients a week to produce enough income to support his growing family. I asked what he was doing to generate income and Patients. He grinned again, this time rather sheepishly, and shrugged his shoulders. "Waiting," he said. At least, I remember thinking, he has a goal.

During the next 18 months of "business surgery," my consulting staff and I were able to put my friend's brother through both a personalized assertiveness training program and then a basic start-up practice management training program. We decorated his office and waiting area, including the infusion of live plants, soft music, carpeting and a small library of related books. We hired an experienced receptionist, and designed and printed business and appointment cards, letterhead, envelopes, and invoices.

We also set up a bookkeeping and collections system, arranged credit and equipment financing (including the price of a permanent, professional examination table), designed and prepared respectable office signs, developed Patient History and Patient Attitude Survey forms, ordered, framed, and hung some appropriate posters, and set up a Patients' Information Bulletin Board.

Next we produced a script and flip chart for public presentations. We got the doctor signed into a public speaking course, booked a series of talks with appropriate local audiences, then wrote and distributed (and arranged placement for) a series of news releases and captioned photos which publicized each of the presentations he gave. We wrote and designed specialty-specific educational materials for him to hand out as part of his presentations. We wrote, designed, and distributed a newsletter, counseled him on how to talk and listen and sit and stand and walk and shake hands, and how to translate his newfound assertiveness and public speaking skills into working with Patients and Patient families. We even devised TelePrompTer-style note cards with key statements for him to refer to when meeting with new Patients. We coached him extensively on his telephone skills. We referred almost all of his first three dozen Patients.

After 18 months, starting from zero, the doctor was seeing forty-nine Patients a week. And 18 months later, after conscientiously following the plans we helped him develop, which included computerizing, expanding his staff and services, and relocating to a medical building, he was seeing thirty Patients a day — at more than three times the rates of the day we first met!

What was the secret? Why couldn't his family succeed at motivating him? What made him appear to be an overnight success? What can you gain and apply from this story, even if your practice is well established?

First, you must be open-minded and receptive to input from the professional resources you take into your confidence. Odds are there is a wealth of experience you can absorb if you're willing to abandon the need to feel "in control." When you let go of this compulsive need, you gain the opportunity to grow. The young doctor in the example cited above listened and absorbed and responded. He valued the input and coaching and worked with it, instead of against it.

Second, the doctor in the example used "Quiet Medical Marketing." He didn't need to run large, blasting, expensive newspaper ads (as his retailer brother suggested). He didn't have to do local radio and TV commercials (as his star-struck mother urged). He didn't need to take a side job in construction "until things get going" (as his father repeatedly and vociferously suggested). He didn't have to outdo his competition who were spending many thousands of dollars on direct mail bombardments. What he needed to do (and did) was to "come alive" by marketing his medical services "quietly," to potential referral sources and to *target* population and geographic groups.

Our most important service to him was not unlike the dynamics of the services that you might provide to a Patient. We assisted with the process of gathering and sorting out information, with preparing a "business diagnosis," with establishing a "professional" (practice and personal) "treatment plan," and with motivating him to follow through with the recommendations. What he learned was that all he had to do, in addition to keeping informed of the latest advances in his field of specialization, was to treat every single Patient and staff contact as the most important one of his life. There can be no more effective marketing for any doctor.

Empathy Breeds Confidence, Trust, and Control

If accepting that notion is difficult for you, you may want to examine your motives for feeling the way you do. Chances are you're really struggling to maintain some sense of personal control. If this is true, you may want to consider that true control is something you can exercise by seeing each Patient and staff encounter as an opportunity to win over the other person's confidence.

Confidence is the cornerstone of trust. If you can't instill some sense of trust in others, you should quit medicine today. Take up basket weaving or become a hermit. How much trust you can earn will determine how successful you can be. Make it your goal to have other people walk away with a sense that you have listened carefully, actively, and attentively to what they had to say. Make it your goal to respond (instead of react) to input from others. Make it your goal to ask productive questions. Make it your goal to take the extra effort to paraphrase what others say.

When you listen and respond and ask questions and paraphrase, and periodically nod your head as you jot down others' comments, you actively demonstrate attentiveness and interest. Think about it. What are the two things you most crave from others when you open your mouth to speak? Odds are 99 out of 100 that your answers are attentiveness and interest. When you take the extra effort to ask Patients, staff, and associates for examples of points they make that are not transparently clear, you ensure more accurate communications.

When you do all these kinds of things, and do them consistently, you begin to gain other people's confidence and, ultimately, their trust. Gaining trust is gaining control at the highest possible level. But trust is inseparably bonded to responsibility. Once you've gained someone's trust, you must also take responsibility for the relationship. You should be prepared to maintain that responsibility for the long haul. Anything less, and you're fooling yourself; you're not in control, you have not gained trust.

The most effective, people-smart doctors we know are those who view their first encounter with every new Patient as an opportunity to build a lifelong relationship, especially when the Patient is someone the doctor would never dream of befriending under any other circumstances. Those Patients who are the most difficult to relate to represent the greatest challenge to your commitment for growth for your self and your practice. They also tend to be those from whom you will reap the greatest referral rewards.

Effective, people-smart doctors focus on more than first time Patients. They zero in on every encounter with every Patient every day. This is work, and considering your clinical responsibilities, it may seem to be a low priority or even frivolous. But reality dictates that Patients can no longer be treated for physical ailments without regard for the nonphysical contributing factors. Regardless of your specialty, you are a doctor of medicine for the whole person. You cannot treat, or even understand the whole person without embracing at least some part of each Patient's personality or probing each lifestyle.

When you think you can't, you can. Look more open-mindedly at others who seek you out. If you don't like someone's face or body or attitude, be more receptive to the possibility that you could learn something from him or her. After all, as truth will have it, the odds are that you are not quite so all-knowing as society would have us believe, and you really haven't walked in someone else's moccasins as often as it might seem.

VI

SCRUB FOR HAPPINESS

Here are two thoughts worthy of your total concentration and ongoing consideration (for at least a few days):

"There is no way to happiness. Happiness is the way." — from *Handbook to Higher Consciousness* (Living Love Center, Berkeley, CA, 1973) by Ken Keyes, Jr.; and

"Happiness Is A Choice" — from the title of the book *Happiness Is A Choice* (Ballantine Books, New York. 1991) by Barry Neil Kaufman.

How can you head home to see your family, or to the office or hospital to see your staff, associates, or Patients, in a good mood and thinking happy thoughts and feeling happy feelings, after arguing with your husband (wife, parent, child, associate), or after learning of a frivolous lawsuit against you, or after having a relative or close friend pass away? How can you be happy after spending all your working hours surrounded by depressed, dispirited, ailing, aching, bitching, moaning, worrying people? How can you swim positively in a sea of negativity? Here are some ideas:

1. *Choose to stop seeing the sea as negative.* Click that mental "radio station" in your head from "24-hour news" (which is always negative) to "easy listening music." Remember, nobody *else* controls *your* "stations" or "channel selector" or "tone" and "Volume" settings.

2. *Choose to experience the "negative people" in your life as "needy"* instead of "negative." Think of them simply as people who need and are waiting for some positive sign from you; a word, a look, a touch that encourages, that reassures. It might only take one positive sign from you for them to become positive themselves. They have a need to think and feel more positive. You have the power.

3. *Fix your sights on "here and now."* Take some deep breaths and pay attention to what's right in front of you with each passing moment. Put the past (more than one minute ago) and future (more than one minute from now) events back into the intangible world they came from.

Sure, it may be "real" that a friend just died, or that you've just been notified of a lawsuit against you, but you can't let the negativity of those things affect your "here and now." They have either passed out of the "here and now," in which case there's nothing you can do about them, or they are part of the uncertain future, which may not even come, and over which — once you have planned for it — you have no other control. The more you mentally key into past and future events, the more you lose your all-important "here and now," and the greater the risk you run of driving into a tree while you're mulling over some 10-minute, 10-hour, or 10-day-old argument, or worrying about some situation that hasn't happened yet, and indeed may never occur. In fact, any personal screw-ups you may have experienced in your private or professional life probably happened because you were not paying 100% attention to what you were doing at the time. Easy to say, you say? Perhaps, but being fully attentive to your unfolding "present" *is* a choice.

4. *Every time you scrub up, use the occasion to make it a mental ritual* of "washing away" all ill feelings and past moments; a preparation for the next "here and now," a self-renewal break, a chance to take a deep breath and clear away all other agenda.

Exercise the same renewal process as you wash your hands before dinner in preparation for your family's "here and now." One doctor has instructed his nurse (and his wife) to remind him to "scrub" whenever he starts to look or act edgy. When actual washing is untimely or impractical, he rubs his hands together briskly, before moving on to the next situation. "Sometimes," he says, "just the thought of it, just being reminded, is enough to calm me down."

5. *Listen to positive music*: "Happy Days Are Here Again," "When You're Smiling, When You're Smiling, The Whole World Smiles With You," "Happy Happy Talk In Happy Town, Talk About Things You Like To Do," "The Happy Whistler," "When Irish Eyes Are Smiling," "Cheer Up, Cheer Up, Get Out Of Bed, Live Life, Love And Be Happy," "Just Put On A Happy Face," etc.

Sing it. Hum it. Whistle it. Program it into your sound system. It's just as easy to listen to music that makes you feel happy as it is to listen to music that makes you feel sad (about 98% of all lyrics?). Just make the choice.

6. *Try reciting aloud this (five or six-second) present tense goal statement*, repeatedly, as you walk, as you exercise, in time to your movements: *"I am relaxed, happy, alert, safe and sound, healthy, wealthy, pain-free, clear (emotionally), 160 (insert desired weight), and physically fit."*

Here are a few helpful hints on how to make this statement work effectively for you: 1) Adapt the statement to your own goals, your own stride, pace or movements; 2) Use it instead of counting numbers — if you normally count to 30, for example, as you stretch, recite this instead five or six times; 3) Say it to yourself as you exhale when you're doing your deep breathing exercises.

The following poem was published in a private book collection entitled *Life Is A Moody Rainbow* (Palomar Press, 1972):

Myself

I

am

delirious,

deciduous,

delighted with myself.

I

am

expended,

extended,

excited with myself

because

I

am,

at last

I've found,

what I am...

I

am

myself.

VII

HOW NOT TO GET KILLED BY SALESPEOPLE

The secret here is in knowing that, to a salesperson, the word "No" means "Yes," and that when you give a reason why you don't want to buy something, you are giving the salesperson the key he or she needs to be able to lock up the sale and walk off with your money.

You did your homework to get your degree, to become certified, to start a practice. You do your homework before tackling a unique or unusual case. Yet, you probably refuse to do any homework when it comes to protecting the very same money you worked so hard to earn. It is transparently clear that a great many doctors are "money - management-illiterate," so if you count yourself among the commonly ripped-off, don't feel too bad. If it's any consolation, remind yourself that hundreds of people around you every day don't have the skills, intelligence, stick-to-itiveness and good fortune to have earned your credentials, and possess your earning power. You are, what most people in our society would term a financial success. Probabilities are, paradoxically, that you are also a money management disaster.

Money, Money, Everywhere, But Not A Drop To Spend

Dr. Redink is a hard-working physician with a one-man band medical practice. He and his support staff had been bringing in nearly $100,000 per day, five days a week, all year long, for a number of years. Yet Dr. Redink was rarely able to afford to buy his own lunches.

Having to declare double bankruptcy shortly after getting started in practice, he learned early on that he had no financial skills. After his debacle, he acted quickly to shore up his money management with the help of an experienced financial officer, whom he hired for a yearly salary of $150,000. How could he go wrong with this set-up? This was, after all, less than two days worth of Patient revenue.

Under a collection of other practice names, created by the

experienced, $150,000-a-year financial officer, the doctor has, at last count, added four more bankruptcies to his credit, or lack thereof. The trail of unpaid bills left in the bankruptcy dust has finally obscured Dr. Redink's image to the point of costing him Patient flow, referrals, income, and sadly, a wife and family who crumbled away under the constant financial pressures.

Moral of the Story: If you're not completely sure of how to manage money, be completely sure that you can be completely sure of the person who manages your money for you. In the instance cited, the doctor tried to rush a solution without doing and homework. He never bothered to check out the "experienced" financial officer. If he did, he would have learned that the man was "experienced" at *bankruptcies* (including two of his own and three of the companies he had run) and that the man also had a reputation among area bankers and lawyers as being rather unscrupulous.

The doctor also failed to communicate clearly to his staff and family that he needed their support, presumably because to do so would have cost him "ego points" by forcing him to acknowledge his personal weaknesses in dealing with money, and by forcing him to own up to his wife that she couldn't have as much money to spend as she had become accustomed to spending.

When it comes time for having excess cash to retire, or fund college educations, or help stabilize a family emergency, you don't want to be in the position of wishing you had been more careful in planning and handling your money, or that you had not been so carefree with your spending habits, or that you had picked a more qualified financial advisor. By then, it's too late.

The time to start dealing more effectively and efficiently with money is now. Today. Practice by doing some homework on the next salesperson, or the next enticing sales phone call, or sales promotion mailing that reaches you. Let whatever the circumstance (regardless of product or service offered) become your target for doing a mini-version of what corporate managers refer to as a "needs assessment" and "feasibility study." You will find the time for this. You'll make the time. If you can't afford the time, you may not be able to afford the price of failing to do the homework. At the very least, find someone you trust to study the sales pitch for you and give you a detailed summary and recommendation of the presentation as well as the quality of the product(s)/service(s) offered, realistic dollar value, and realistic extent of need.

Be Careful of "Harmless" Questions

One short example of a popular sales technique for making, or "closing" a sale is to get the prospect (that's you!) to respond positively to a minor "either/or" question: "If you were to buy this Porsche, Dr. Impresyerfrends, would you prefer your initials on the door panels to be in gold or in silver?" After answering a few of these subordinate inquiries (and becoming preoccupied with relatively insignificant issues) with the salesperson recording your responses directly onto the order form, signing the dotted line doesn't feel difficult at all. In the process of making minor commitments, it becomes an unspoken understanding that you've already committed to purchasing the car. After all, by signing off, you're just confirming a bunch of little decisions, and (heaven knows) you really would look terrific behind the wheel. Happy payments!

A better way to handle the situation is simply to not answer questions. Instead, say: "Thank you for your interest in my preferences, but if I decide to buy a car here, I'll buy it, and at that time I'll let you know exactly what I want." Or, "I'm the customer, how about I ask the questions?"

Picture the following scenario: You have just defeated the X-ray equipment sales representative who has valiantly tried to convince you to upgrade, but you've held your ground and she's now about to leave your office. You start to feel a bit smug with your victory, but little did you know, this rep has undergone advanced tactical combat training. She has mastered, and proceeds to use, the "Columbo Technique." Following her "failed" sales effort, she gets to your door, opens it, smiles and offers some parting pleasantries. She steps out through your doorway as you sigh in relief, and almost pulls the door completely closed. But then, just before the latch clicks shut, she leans back into your office (just like Peter Falk does as television Detective Columbo with a freshly-questioned suspect) and says, "By the way, Doc, now that we've agreed you're not buying, would you mind telling me the *real* reason you don't want to upgrade?"

You respond with some feeble half-truth, and she meanders back in to the edge of your desk with a whole new, much more focused sales effort that nails down your "real reason" with irrefutable logic. Does any of this sound familiar?

In the personal-growth-through-outdoor-adventure company, Outward Bound, one of the program instructors reportedly lectured participants on the reality of stress factors during the "Solo" period, wherein each individual is left alone to survive in the wilderness for 24 hours with nothing but a knife): "When you feel butterflies in your stomach," she advised the participants, "don't try to chase them away; teach them to fly in formation."

When you feel overwhelmed by salespeople, don't waste energy trying to chase them away; teach them to work for you. Detail reps can be valuable to you in terms of doing research for you or teaching you about new products and procedures. And they're not the only ones who can help you this way. Try asking other kinds of salespeople (regardless of the product or service they represent...cameras, insurance, stocks and bonds, real estate, surgical equipment, stereos, cars, office supplies, etc.) lots of questions.

Pretend the product or service you're considering or shopping for is a new Patient who can only respond through it's parent, the salesperson. Ask and then listen. Believe it or not, salespeople are people too. And they love to teach if you'll just give them the chance. Keep in mind that salespeople also need (and appreciate your help) to determine if you are a "prospect" or a "suspect." ["suspects" window-shop, "kick tires," and often never buy; "prospects" usually become "customers."]

In the same fashion you would want a definitive answer from a Patient about proceeding with a complex treatment plan, good salespeople would rather have a definite "no" than a "maybe," and will appreciate, just like you, not having their time wasted.

Those salespeople who push their wares, their messages, or themselves to the point that you feel uncomfortable, are probably not the kinds of people you want to deal with anyway. Simply send them on their merry way, regardless of how sophisticated or credentialed they seem to be, and regardless of who referred them to you. They're wasting your time.

Theater producer David Belasco reportedly told solicitors that if they could write their idea on the back of their business card, he would consider seeing them. [I tried this for awhile with walk-in-off-the-street salespeople; almost all would quietly leave within 30 seconds of hearing the challenge!] A busy west coast doctor plunks a 3-minute egg timer down on her desk for every sales call, as a measure of maximum time allowed for a salesperson to "get to the point" of each visit, before getting a request to leave. "Most of them waste no time, and the good reps enjoy rising to the occasion, which, of course," she says, "I enjoy too!" In this way, the doctor adds, when she spends longer time periods with sales reps, it's *her* choice, not theirs.

Enlightened Self-Interest

The overall rule of thumb for how not to get killed by salespeople is to view every practice-related purchase decision (including, and especially those related to marketing and community involvement) as needing to fit under the umbrella of "Enlightened Self-Interest." Ask yourself if the expense involved has direct bearing on being "Enlightened" as to the needs of your Patients, your staff, or your referrers. Think of the "S" in "Self" as a "$," and the "I" in "Interest" as standing for "Investment."

Buying a full page of advertising space in a fund-raising journal for a single men's bowling league tournament, or serving as on-field physician for the neighborhood high school football team may be appropriate for a sports medicine practice, but hardly makes sense for an OB/GYN. Don't take this as insultingly basic stuff. I recently spotted a pediatrician with a display booth at a senior citizens health fair. When I asked him why he was there, he replied in a very matter-of-fact tone, "to influence grandparents to bring their grandchildren to me." His time would have been better spent addressing a children's class, a PTA meeting, or a new mothers' support group.

Measure each decision against the question of what potential return there could possibly be. If it's not worth it, it's not worth it. *Bottom Line*: It's just as easy and just as responsible (and much more rewarding) to be a "do-gooder" for crusades, causes, and public events that can provide some potential form of payback to your practice, as it is to be a "do-gooder" for something that bears no possible return on investment to your practice or community image.

Be Careful of "Pyramid Marketing" Schemes

I've been to doctors' homes when they've hosted pyramid marketing company sales and recruitment presentations to other doctors for some very fine quality products and services. The people making the presentations have been very polished, highly communicative, and extremely engaging. The presentation materials (charts, graphs, signs, handouts, etc.) have been professionally produced and very cleverly explained. The systems they have represented for making money have usually been oversimplified and overrated. In the end, these systems always depend on each "investor" to cultivate highly motivated people, who will cultivate highly motivated people, who will cultivate highly motivated people.

While these "investment plans" are not always illegal, they are, at the very least, horribly deceptive. Companies that sell their products or services in any kind of a process that reminds you of how a chain letter works, are not worth one minute of your time or one dollar from your wallet. Period.

Since most pyramid-type organizations are so dependent on referrals of motivated people, they often become a breeding ground for those who are involved to "recruit" friends and family members, often under the guise of doing them "favors." This brings us to the subject of how and when to say "No" to financial proposals from friends, associates and family members.

Assertiveness, i.e., having a well-developed skill for saying "Yes" and "No," regardless of the person making the proposal, is critical to financial survival for every doctor.

At this point, you may be pondering the following question: "How can I turn down people who are close to me? Saying no is different when I'm asked to invest money with, or loan money to, my brother or sister or cousin or associate or neighbor. Having a reputation for being cheap is not how I want to be known to friends and family."

The answer? Responding to an investment or loan request with a "yes" does not mean "Yes, I love you." Responding with a "No" does not mean "No, I don't love you." Stop equating your rejection of a financial request from someone you care about with no longer caring about that person. If, on a consistent basis, you don't view things that way, others, over time, won't either.

If you use the right words, people will understand your rationale. Simply say: "I love you very much, dear brother (or other relative), and I support your efforts to do A, B, and C, but the method I have set up for investing money simply doesn't allow for me to make any hasty decisions; it also doesn't allow me to make them without consulting someone."

"I would love to be able to afford to make you an interest-free loan, or great neighbor of mine, but I can't. I do consider you to be an important person in my life, but you need to know that I consider any loan to be a business arrangement. I am willing, therefore, to do the next best thing, which is to offer you better terms than the bank offers (lower interest rate, or lower payments spread out over a longer period, or no collateral, etc.) in exchange for your signed and notarized promissory note."

"I don't normally do this, my esteemed colleague, but if you're willing to meet with my accountant, lawyer, and financial advisor — the people I've given responsibility to for deciding on my investments — to answer their questions and outline all the details of what you had in mind, I'll go along with their recommendations."

For smaller amounts of money, the answer is simple: if it's not in your pocket, you can't take it out of your pocket to give to someone. Make a practice of not carrying any more cash than you need for a day's worth of food, coffee, etc., or at least make a practice of not showing it. Depending on office and hospital neighborhoods frequented, many doctors keep their wallets locked up or hidden in their cars, instead of lying around in a briefcase, pocketbook, or discarded jacket as they tend to their patients.

VIII

GIMMICKS, GADGETS, AND OTHER EGO-TRIP RIP-OFFS

"Now that you mention it, we could really use some advice on marketing. We've spent an awful lot of money on stuff that didn't work," said the diagnostic facility's vice president of operations. "We absolutely have," I was reassured by the medical director, a cardiologist. Perhaps I looked a bit skeptical. At any rate, the other partner, a pulmonist, chimed in, "They're not kidding! We have a whole closet full of stuff. You wouldn't believe it!"

The VP promptly slid his chair back from our meeting table, strode across the room, and disappeared through a doorway adjacent to his desk. The two doctors stared blankly at each other for the next minute or so, and then the VP suddenly reappeared with a huge, filled-to-the-brim shopping bag that he dumped upside down on the conference table.

Out tumbled executive umbrellas with the facility's logo, ceramic tiles (for coffee mug desk protection!) with the facility's logo, coffee mugs (of course!) with their logo, T-shirts with their logo, along with logo-imprinted key chains, rulers, magnets, even lollipops. You name it, they had it. I was tempted to ask the pulmonist if they had had any ashtrays made up, but decided to keep my tongue in my cheek.

Clearly, an alert salesperson saw the opportunity to strike at their naive throats, and was able to walk off with a hefty commission (and, no doubt, a laugh up his or her sleeve as well).

And so, the VP and two doctor/directors began a discussion that morning that quickly became an abbreviated version of "You Learn From Your Mistakes 101." They were able to put their collection of "advertising specialty" rip-off items in proper perspective. In the process of looking at and handling the various products, they gained some insight about how purchasing items like these couldn't really be considered "marketing" or "advertising." In fact, given the facility's primary target of corporate personnel and risk managers (to arrange executive health exams), these items did not even constitute common sense selections.

Increases in Patient volume finally came with a shift in marketing emphasis from gimmicks and newspaper ads to personal, one-on-one sales calls that emphasized quality and convenience of service. The establishment of a tightly controlled budget that preempted whimsical purchases (logo imprint-type items) also played a major role in this area. For some doctors, imprinted junk is addictive.

"Pocket-Money Suicide"

Many doctors slowly "kill" themselves financially by consistently thinking that spending only "pocket change" or "petty cash" (any amount around or less than $100) for imprinted pens, stickers, key rings, etc. is no big deal. And the truth is, it's not. Once or twice. But some doctors can't stop at once or twice. One New York firm specializing in imprinted novelty items, reports numerous doctor/customers who place "regular" orders for "a few hundred dollars *a month*."

If you have a deep-seated need to "see your name up in lights" on every passing piece of plastic, glass, metal, ceramic, rubber or whatever, go ahead and indulge yourself. Get it out of your system, but be aware that "ego expenses" are never likely to result in a logjam in your Patient appointment book.

Now, is it true that most doctors tend to be suckers for gimmicks and gadgets? Absolutely. What about all the contraptions and devices you've filed patent applications for, or considered (or actually tried) inventing over the years? How many "doctoring" instruments do you own that you never use, and don't really need? How many times have you gotten "lost" in a home center or hardware store, and ended up with a garage or workbench or "junk drawer" full of oddball tools that you probably never even pick up? Close your eyes for ten seconds and think about that.

Gadgets and gimmicks do get doctors' attention and interest. Sometimes, "just the right" gadget or gimmick, accompanied by "just the right" message, and distributed in "just the right" way to other doctors, can help soften or establish relations, and open the door to a strengthened referral base.

Speaking of "Opening Doors..."

"Not too long ago, a combination like this was state-of-the-art for tooth removal!," read the tag, tied with a three-foot piece of string to an old doorknob. This item was mailed to dentists by an oral surgeon seeking

new referrals in a highly competitive market. The tag opened into a small folder that emphasized the oral surgeon's modern equipment, 24-hour availability, nurturing staff, and commitment to maintaining a strong partnership communication level with each referring dentist. Each doorknob had the oral surgeon's name and phone number printed on it.

Twelve out of 16 dentists contacted responded with phone calls complimenting the mailing. One even sent back an old pair of pliers, suggesting the string and doorknob left too much to chance. The oral surgeon now enjoys ongoing Patient referrals from five dentists he didn't know before.

An M.D. specialist in nutritional medicine who was struggling to gain area acceptance and referrals from "mainstream" primary care providers, found success with hand-deliveries of gift-wrapped pickles with notes that read: "Odds are that many of your patients think they are getting their green vegetables every day by eating slices of this on their hamburgers, or chunks of it on their hot dogs. As a result, I am in something of a pickle myself right now, and could use your help... Can I buy you the rest of lunch next week so I can explain how we might work together, Dr. Familyman, for the benefit of your patients who have eating disorders? My assistant will call your office Wednesday to arrange a date. I look forward to seeing you. Regards, Dr. Healthnut."

Here are some enterprising approaches from an ophthalmologist we'll call Dr. Mack D'generayshun, who decided to tackle two of the most productive potential sources for referrals any doctor could have: 1) other doctors (in this case, optometrists); and 2) existing Patients. Dr. D'generayshun arranged for hand-delivery of clear, "see-through" telephones, to every optometrist listed in his phone directory. Each phone sported personalized, engraved bronze plates that looked something like this:

**DR. EYEGUY'S
EYE HEALTH HOT LINE**
TO MACK D'GENERAYSHUN, M.D. F.A.A.O.
020-020-2020

Hanging out from inside each window-boxed telephone (by a 12-inch piece of hemp tied to the phone cord) were two personalized, typeset, hole-punched tags that were printed on fluorescent-colored paper and glued to cardboard. These Tags are shown in Figures 8-1 and 8-2. Front desk staff people were instructed to not put any "Hot Line" calls on hold, and to be sure that any incoming optometrist calls would be connected directly with their doctor (or when that wasn't practical, to interrupt the practice manager).

Notice the double entendre use of "see through." Advertising copywriters have long known that headlines with double meanings are more memorable, and often more provocative ("Does She, Or Doesn't She? Only Her Hairdresser Knows For Sure," for Clairol haircoloring, and "The Dog Kids Love To Bite," for Armour Hot Dogs, are classic examples).

To avoid any potential problems with medical board regulations on gift-giving (and because it makes good charitable, community-image sense), the hand-printed "P.S." at the bottom of Figure 8-2 was added to highlight and personalize the suggestion to donate the phone.

The "Honesty..." theme line at the bottom of the large tag is a carryover from the doctor's newspaper ads that emphasized the point in an attempt to "play up" his high sense of ethics, at a time when some other Ophthalmologists in the area had been getting a considerable amount of bad publicity for doing "unnecessary" surgery and for "overcharging" on office visits and procedures.

Why go to such extravagant lengths on a promotional item of this type? Because many doctors like to see their names set in type or engraved in metal. Personalization always gets a response. Why go to all of this trouble just to prompt a lunch? The personalized telephone and personalized attention break the ice for a lunch invitation that would otherwise seem awkward, and would be less likely to gain a receptive ear. And Dr. D'generayshun, in addition to being a skilled surgeon, is also a gifted and engaging joke-teller.

A get-to-know-you-lunch meeting, peppered with smiles and a laugh or two, may seem like a shallow reason to consider referring Patients. But reality is that, outside of rural, small town settings, very few professionals ever take the time and trouble to get acquainted personally with one of their most important referral resources and referral prospects — other professionals. So whoever does take the time and trouble, and continues to do so with some regularity (even a breakfast meeting or round of golf two or three times a year), usually gets the lion's share of new Patients.

Dr. D'generayshun succeeded at establishing some strong, new working relationships with a number of area optometrists (who also, not

Figure 8-1

NOW YOU CAN "SEE THROUGH" EVERY PATIENT CALL FROM BEGINNING TO END, DR. EYEGUY...

With this *Eye Health Hotline* phone, and Dr. D'generayshun as your *On-Call Consultant and Surgeon,* you can *"see"* your Patients *"through"* every step of testing and care.

You can follow the progress for each — from diagnosis or diagnostic confirmation to prognosis, treatment and followup — and never lose sight of them because:

1. **YOU KEEP YOUR PATIENTS** for all their normal eyecare needs. This we guarantee. We color-code our files to be absolutely sure that your patients remain your patients at all times.

2. **YOU GET PRIORITY UPDATES** for every patient you send us, whether it's for surgery or just a consulting opinion. Our comprehensive updates are provided according to *your* scheduling needs.

3. **YOU CONTROL CATARACT POST-OPERATIVE VISITS** if you wish, and bill accordingly. Dr. D'generayshun will see your patients the day and week following surgery. If all's well, they can return to you for other visits.

4. **YOU CAN CONFIDENTLY PROVIDE PATIENTS WITH A MEDICAL EXPERT** to consult with and assist you in diagnosing and treating any extraordinary eye problems... from glaucoma to ocular tumors.

5. **YOU CAN TAKE ADVANTAGE OF OUR EQUIPMENT RESOURCES** by sending patients for our on-premise Visual Field Testing or treatment with one of our three (in-office) separate laser systems.

6. **YOU ARE WELCOME TO "CO-MANAGE" PATIENTS** with certain eye diseases, such as glaucoma or diabetic retinopathy... just let us know.

7. **YOU CONTINUE TO BE NUMBER ONE FOR CONTACT AND EYEGLASS LENSES,** frames, sunglasses, etc. *Our medical practice is 100% medical.*

We do everything we can to make it easy, convenient and comfortable for each and every patient. We are approved by all insurance carriers, and accept all major credit cards

We are committed to making each Patient you send to our office... for cataract removal, laser procedures, and specialized consulting or treatment... appreciative of your skills, good judgement and professional resources.

We believe that honest business is good business, especially when it comes to healthcare... doing what makes good sense and being ethical in all of our contacts.

020-020-2020

BIG MAC, INC.
One Cataract Way
Fuzzyvue, NY

MACK D'GENERAYSHUN, M.D., F.A.A.E.S.

A summarized listing of all professional and community affiliations goes in this box. A summarized listing of all professional and community affiliations goes in this box. A summarized listing of all professional and community affiliations goes in this box. A summarized listing of all professional and community affiliations goes in this box.

Figure 8-2

Dear Dr. Eyeguy,

You can test your new phone and "see the light" with a call to our office.
Simply key in the number shown on your nameplate, then announce: "This is a
'Hotline Call' for Dr. D'generayshun." Our front desk staff promises to connect you
directly to me (or my practice manager, Iris).

In return for the courtesy of your call, I'd like to set up a time I can treat you to lunch
so we can discuss some teamwork details. I look forward to hearing from you.

Best Regards,

Mack D'generayshun

Mack D'generayshun, M.D.

P.S. GOT ENOUGH PHONES? AFTER YOU'VE MADE
YOUR LUNCHDATE CALL, YOU MAY WANT TO REMOVE
THE NAMEPLATE (IT'S 2-SIDED-TAPED) SO YOU CAN
DONATE THE PHONE TO A FAVORITE CHARITY. MD

incidentally, are rarely approached by ophthalmologists for anything). In addition, he learned a great deal about the eye healthcare market from a professional retail perspective, which helped him guide his staff to relate more realistically to his Patients.

Orthopaedic surgeons and chiropractors who have exercised the same "getting to know you" dynamics — by making the extra effort to build relationships with lawyers specializing in personal injury cases — consistently outperform other orthopods and other chiropractors in generating increased numbers of patient referrals.

Flower Power

As for Dr. D'generayshun's *Patient* promotion effort, his office launched a highly successful program of distributing fresh, long-stemmed flowers with an attached tag that appears in Figure 8-3. The flowers are delivered fresh, twice a week, in half-filled buckets of water, and tags are fastened by front desk people (between phone calls and clerical tasks), who also distribute them to every man, woman and child who leaves the office; this includes postal and package delivery people, Patient "drivers," friends and family members who accompany Patients, and even visiting sales representatives. If a Patient has to come in two or three times in one week, he or she gets a tagged, fresh flower each time. The 35 cents per flower expense costs far less than traditional advertising or promotion programs, and more than pays for itself in Patient referrals. How is that possible?

Figure 8-3

Thank You **MACK D'GENERAYSHUN, M.D.**
One Cataract Way • Fuzzyvue, NY 02002
020/020-2020

We really appreciate having you as our visitor today. We hope you'll think of Dr. D'generayshun next time someone mentions needing a good eye doctor, eye surgery or treatment, or a general eye exam.

Have a wonderful day! *From Dr. D'generayshun and Staff*

Because the impact of this seemingly small gesture is not to be believed! In addition to satisfied Patients leaving the office feeling even more satisfied, dissatisfied Patients find it hard to stay grumpy and irate while they're standing at your front desk (or headed home) with a live flower in their hands.

Except, perhaps, for an allergist, this idea will work for virtually every kind of medical and healthcare practice or facility. The key to success with this program is to be absolutely sure that the person(s) giving out the flowers act(s) like it's a big deal/special occasion every single time, with every single visitor (and, of course, to make sure that the flowers are always fresh).

There is an additional hidden benefit to this practice. The constant presence of flowers at the front desk, and the process of giving them out, serve as an ongoing morale booster to staff people and can help provide some cheery visual relief to some otherwise stressful job functions. In addition, end-of-the-week leftovers are divided up for the staff to take home on Friday night.

For extra enhancement, try having the involved staff person(s) produce a handmade "Flower Power" poster for your waiting area to help maximize program awareness. The poster can feature a drawing or painting of a long-stemmed carnation (or mum, or whatever flower you select), and have two small holes on either side of the stem (about two-thirds of the way up) to loosely hook (or ribbon tie) an actual flower tag onto the poster. The bottom one-third of the stem can have large-type, bold-face words such as these written over it:

**THANK YOU FOR VISITING OUR OFFICE TODAY.
AS YOU LEAVE, WE HAVE A BEAUTIFUL,
LONG-STEMMED FLOWER FOR YOU TO TAKE HOME.
IT'S OUR WAY OF LETTING YOU KNOW
HOW MUCH WE APPRECIATE YOUR HEALTHCARE TRUST,
AND YOUR REFERRALS TO FRIENDS AND FAMILY.**

Have the poster displayed next to the desk, counter, or window where Patients pay and schedule follow-up appointments.

Stick-to-itiveness

Being aware of the fact that so very many people like to have their name and message on a refrigerator magnet, and that virtually everyone uses them, it's difficult not to admit that these are reasonable promotional items to spend money on. Even with magnets, however, designing them to serve some larger purpose than holding up children's artwork helps justify the expense. "Fold-over" and "clip" style magnets that hold appointment cards are examples of items with more functional promotional value.

Be careful not to underestimate the surprisingly negative impact that some of your imprinted items can have on existing and potential Patients. Things that are, or appear to be, very expensive can cause people to question your fees, your ethics, and your judgement. Things that are, or appear to be, too cheap can cause people to question the quality of your services, your equipment, and your judgement. Things that are inappropriate to your practice can cause people to question the appropriateness of your examinations, tests, treatments and treatment plans.

A Dental implantologist came to be known locally as "The Apple Dentist" with "Take One" bushel baskets of apples on his office counter, and even in his van for offerings at his son's soccer games. His ads, newsletters, and business and appointment reminder cards all sport an apple missing a big bite, accompanied by the words, "Yes, You Can..."

A midwest pediatrician hands out imprint-wrapper-covered, sugar-free, "safety" lollipops to her Patients and to her Patient's parents.

A mobile unit veterinarian who travels extensively between distant farms gives Patient owners a red-painted horseshoe with his name and phone number hand-printed in white across the face. Most of these get hung up near the phone, or over barn or kitchen doorways.

Cardiac rehab Patients receive health food store discount coupons and "Have A Heart" sweatshirts. What's wrong with all this? Nothing. In each instance, the item involved is something that relates directly to the nature of the care provided and, on the receiving end, is generally considered to be a nice personal touch, symbolic to many of a friendly, caring doctor.

IX

DIRECT MARKETING

How and When You Say What You Say Says It All

While most doctors will readily admit that marketing probably makes use of some mysterious manner and degree of "art," there are a good many traditionalist, highbrow types who take offense at even the suggestion that "science" (being so "pure") could possibly be involved with something so crude and tainted and distasteful as marketing.

The fact is that effective marketing, and especially *direct* marketing (because it's the most measurable form of marketing), is a remarkably sophisticated blend of simplistic creativity and carefully analyzed test results — both art and science. The problem most nonmarketing people have with recognizing and appreciating this is that there isn't a whole lot of effective marketing going on to begin with, least of all in healthcare.

"Hurry, Hurry, Step Right Up..."

It's 8:15 on a typical Sunday evening. The household has settled into the standard end-of-the-weekend coma. The dog is curled up under a corner table, one eye partially open. The kids are playing "quietly" upstairs. Mom is finally sitting with her feet up, watching some no-brainer movie of the week. And Dad has sunken half out of sight into his lounge chair, almost asleep under what looks like two trees worth of Sunday newspaper. The weekend has been fast-paced, fun, and tiring for all. These last few peaceful moments before bedtime seem precious indeed. Suddenly, the tranquil scene is pierced by the shrill ring of the telephone.

Ring, ring, ring!
Bark, bark, bark, bark!
Ring, ring, ring!

Dad: "Would someone please get that?"

Ring, ring, ring!

Bark, bark, bark, bark!

Ring, ring, ring!

Dad: "Please?!"

Ring, ring, ring!

Bark, bark, bark, bark!

Ring, ring, ring!

Dad: "Oh, never mind, I'll get it! (pause) Hello?"

Salesman: "Hi, Mr. Peaceandquiet? (no pause) How are you today? (no pause) This is Crackauback Chiropractic Center calling to tell you about our Super Special Spine Subluxation Service. (quick breath) For just $19.95, you and one member of your family can take advantage of our comprehensive Crackauback Chiropractic Center examination/treatment/x-ray package deal, with Dr. Digswithfist or Dr. Pipewrench. (quick breath) Can we schedule you for next Tuesday morning or would Tuesday afternoon be better?"

Dad: "Oh sure, you can do that. Tuesday, huh? Yeah, the afternoon is great! Write me down."

Salesman: "That's very good, sir. Is three o'clock ok?"

Dad: "Fantastic!"

Salesman: "Very good, sir (sounding pleased with himself). And who in your family will you be bringing along?"

Dad: "Sam."

Salesman: "Sam?"

Dad: "Sam."

Salesman: "That's your son, sir?"

Dad: "No, that's my cocker spaniel. He pulled a back muscle just now when the ringing phone startled him and he jumped up and hit the bottom of the table he was lying under. And why was he so rattled about some little old telephone rings, you ask? Because even a *dog* knows that only a total idiot would be calling us at home, at 8:15 on a Sunday night, to try to promote a professional service like you were selling vacuum cleaners. Good night, Mr. Screwloose!"

Effective telemarketing, textbooks say, requires the use of "Diagram" or "If" scripts that show the caller what to say in every situation, in answer to every conceivable type of response. Here's an example of an "If" script used to follow up target mailings from an orthopaedic surgeon soliciting referrals from "P.I." (Personal Injury) lawyers:

[Reminders: Sit up straight and smile (use the mirror in front of you as a reminder), both posture and smiles can be "heard." Take a deep breath before and after each call. Remember that, to anyone you speak with, you are not just *representing* Chainsaw Orthopaedics, you *are* Chainsaw Orthopaedics.]

You say: "Good morning/afternoon. This is Chainsaw Orthopaedics calling for Mr./Ms./Mrs. (insert lawyer's last name). I have a quick question to ask him/her for Dr. Chainsaw. Is he/she available right now?"
If you hear: "Yes" or "I'll connect you" or "I'll check..."
You say: "That's great, thank you very much." *And proceed to* *
If you hear: "No" or "I'll take the message" or "He/she is out/in a meeting/away from the desk/in court/very busy,..."
You say: "Okay, well, Dr. Chainsaw really wants me to ask the question directly, and not **leave** a message, but I'd be happy to try back if you could please tell me when you think would be the best time to call. I'll only need about a minute and a half with him/her."
If you hear: No response.
You say: "So what time do you suggest would be the most likely time to reach him/her?" [When you get a response, repeat back the exact time suggested in the form of a question. "Do I understand you correctly that we should try calling back between _____ and _____?" When it's confirmed, write it down. Be sure to call back at the exact time.] "Thank you. Have a great day/afternoon/evening!"

* "Hi, Mr./Ms./Mrs. _____, this is Chainsaw Orthopaedics calling. My name is _____ (first name only). Dr. Chainsaw asked me to contact you to find out if you received the letter and brochure he mailed you last/this week, and, related to that, if you have any ideas for him that might help to strengthen the relationship of his practice with your firm. He's especially interested in having your thoughts about fee structure for legal reports in P.I. and worker's comp cases." [Write down any response offered.]

[If the person you're speaking with says he or she never received the mailing, or wants another, ask how you might best address it to make sure he/she gets it, and write down whatever is said. Then proceed to prompt for an answer to the second half of your question (...if you have any ideas for him...") and write down any response offered before proceeding to ** and ***.]

** "Thank you very much for your time and comments, Mr./Ms./Mrs. _____. I'll be sure that Dr. Chainsaw gets your input. Will it be okay for him to call you back if he has any questions?" [Write down any response.]

[*Special Note*: If at any time the person you are calling interrupts you, be sure to make written notes of what he/she says, and be sure to get back to completing the full script. Be prepared to discuss Dr. Chainsaw's background (refer to a biographical information sheet). It is extremely important to write down every statement or comment made.]

*** "Our number here at Chainsaw Orthopaedics is 1-800-BUZ-ZZZZ. Any time you call, please identify yourself as an attorney. Our switchboard/receptionist/ front desk staff has instructions to handle attorney calls to Chainsaw Orthopaedics as a priority. Thanks again, Mr./Ms./Mrs. _____, and have a nice day/afternoon/evening."

Effective telemarketing, the textbooks say, requires that callers use headsets and a mirror to make their calls. Headsets are used so hands are free to move and enhance voice expression, to take notes more easily, to ensure greater concentration, to prevent sore necks and shoulders, and to encourage better posture, which is reflected in voice delivery. Mirrors are used to look into during calls, to monitor posture and smiles. Both really *can* be "heard."

[This ability of people to "hear" visual actions is a critically important point to keep in mind when you are teleconferencing Patients or other professionals who, reasonably or not, will judge much of what you say by how clearly and pleasantly you say it.]

Textbooks aside, however, experience and reality dictate that healthcare telemarketing is a very delicate exercise, and when necessary, it is best done by you and your staff personally, and without scripts! An informal, sincere and empathetic approach will do just fine. Absolutely nothing has more positive impression values than the doctor herself or himself making direct phone calls to a post-op or past visit Patient the next day (and the next week!) to check on the Patient's status. (If you haven't the time for this, you're not managing your time properly to begin with. If you believe you are managing your time properly, but still don't have time to make personal follow-up calls, then you simply don't get it; Patients will *respond* to your follow up attention, they will *react* to lack of it!)

As for the prescribed equipment, you'll probably never have enough free time to justify the cost of the headset for your *own* use (unless you've always dreamed of being an air traffic controller or radio call-in talk show host). For anyone making or receiving a large volume of calls in your office, however, headsets can be very effective tools. This is especially tools when multiple tasks — like chart filling and retrieval and/or computer input and retrieval — are called for by the individual(s) handling incoming and outgoing calls.

Mirrors, for any size practice phone-user, are probably not a bad idea. But please leave the cutesy 800 phone number acronyms for hospitals, medical centers, retailers and politicians. They *need* the edge. If you're a good doctor who has, and shows, genuine concern for your Patients, you don't need a 1-800-GOOD-DOC to build and sustain Patient flow volume. The only "edge" you need is to keep doing what you're doing.

A prominent M.D./CEO of a PPO (sounds like "government-speak") had to be practically knocked unconscious by his advisors before he was convinced to give up his idea of a 900 phone number for the public to call his Preferred Provider Organization. At a rate of $5 for the first minute, plus another dollar or two for every minute thereafter, the caller could get comprehensive medical background information for any one of 50 different specialists. Among the many problems with this plan was the fact that it was being proposed in a state with thousands of specialists and free 800 number referral services in abundance, and at a time when 900 exchange phone numbers were being equated with pay-for-phone-sex calls and a wide assortment of less than reputable merchandise offers. Unless this doctor had a disproportionately high percentage of telephone company stock in his portfolio, why he would fight so hard for something so stupid?

Simple. He was being the stereotypical demanding doctor (who, of course, envisioned himself as a sharp businessman, which he was not) with an attitude of "I want what I want, when I want it, no matter what the cost, no matter what anybody else thinks, no matter whether it makes sense or not." A further sampling of this same doctor's approach to direct marketing, which speaks for itself in terms of abundant marketing failures and hundreds of thousands of dollars worth of wasted mailings, is the advice he used to give his advisors in terms of their approach to marketing: "You are always 'Ready, Aim, Fire,' and that's what's wrong with you. I am 'Fire, Aim, Ready,' which is why I always get the jump on other doctors."

Direct marketing is a 100% waste of money, time, and effort if you don't *test, test, test* before implementing a complete program. Doing a major mailing without first trying some sample mailings is like deciding to remove someone's colon, with no diagnostic tests or scans, because of a stomachache complaint.

Scientific measurement of direct mail has been going on since long before television was even invented. Since the 1940s and 50s, office libraries and bookshelves of famous direct mail companies such as Prentice-Hall (then known primarily for textbook and professional newsletter publishing) and Fischer-Stevens (then known primarily for medical mailing list rentals) were packed with literally tens of thousands of reports on the results of tests conducted on every conceivable facet of direct mail solicitations.

Did you know, for example, that envelopes bearing commemorative stamps will always get opened before those with regular stamps, which will always get opened before those with bulk rate stamps, which will always get opened before those with meter imprints, which will always get opened before those with bulk rate meter imprints, etc.? As for envelope addressing, personally handwritten is best. Computer "handwritten" is next best. Personally typed is next, followed by word-processor typed, followed (far behind) by imprinted see-through labels, imprinted labels that are color-coordinated with return address imprints, and white imprinted labels. Addressing mail by name and title is most desirable, by name alone is second best, and by title alone is a distant third.

Mailing lists are available from many sources (local services are better — more accurate and more economical — than major list rental companies; homemade lists from phone books and community organization directories are best). Local individualized mailing services are also better than major mailing service companies, but again, having your own staff do the work is usually the best way to ensure accuracy and economy. When your staff is simply too busy, group and stagger the mailings so ten or twenty pieces go out each day or week. Develop a plan that works best for you and your practice.

The bottom line with direct mail format: the more personal the mailing appears to be, the more likely it will get noticed, opened, considered, and responded to. The bottom line with direct mail content: The more you tell, the more you sell. First class postage (which should *always* be used) covers the cost of four to five standard sheets of paper. Include information pages with your letters and invoices to get your money's worth of postage and enhance your prospects for positive responses. Always include phone numbers and reply cards.

Probably the world's greatest experts in the area of direct marketing are executive recruitment and placement firm representatives. They use highly targeted approaches and continuously cultivated resources. They have a success formula rule of thumb that helps produce a success ratio high above the normal (usually quoted at 1-3%) response rate: "Follow up every letter with a phone call, another letter and another phone call; and follow up every phone call with a letter, another phone call, and another letter."

Keeping in mind that sales studies tell us it takes, on the average, five attempts to "close" a sale, it's not surprising that any strategy based on perseverance will be productive. For effective direct mail efforts, keep the results of this study in mind, and combine them with the two basic premises of all successful sales, advertising, and promotion campaigns: 1) Repetition Sells! Repetition Sells! Repetition Sells!, and 2) Follow Up! Follow Up! Follow Up!

Doctors are no exception, susceptibility-wise, to the impact values of "Repetition Sells" and "Follow Up." Those doctors who are most successful at building strong referral relationships are, themselves, carefully repetitive in the words they use to prompt referrals.

Specialists seeking primary care provider referrals, for example, will want to emphasize referrer benefits, such as: "I/we respect your right and concern to monitor the diagnostic/treatment progress of any patients you refer...I/we will keep you informed on any basis you request, from immediate phone calls and faxes, to short-term summaries, to long-term plan reports."

Where it's appropriate, use words such as: "You are assured that every patient you send us will be directed back to your office for follow-up care as soon as the specialized procedures you sent the patient here for have been completed."

The number of times selected words, such as "your right to monitor" and "directed back to your office," appear in follow-up contacts is critically important. Equally important are the various ways the selected sets of words are communicated. Use all your resources. Convey whatever sets of benefit words you choose consistently — in person, by mail, by fax, by phone, and by messenger. (A messenger carrying a personal, handwritten note — with the right words and coaching — is the next best thing to being there yourself!)

As for budgeting considerations when evaluating direct marketing costs vs. those of other media, be careful not to be trapped by mass media reps (for television, radio, newspaper, magazine, and outdoor billboards) who love to feed your analytical mind a dazzling diet of statistical survey results showing superiority of their particular station, publication, etc. It's easy to be convinced of the dollar efficiency of media advertising when you're presented with figures showing an advertising vehicle's ability to reach three gazillion people for less than one-half penny per day each. Or how you can have a captive audience of forty-nine skillion prospective patients for the amount you would make on just one patient who comes to your office because of the advertisement placed.

There's not a newspaper or radio station sales rep alive that won't jump to show you their market position ratings at the drop of a hat. Ever wonder why? It's because (didn't you know?) everyone is "Number One!" If you can find a media sales rep who tells you her or his publication or station is 4th or 3rd, or even 2nd in the marketplace, it probably means that you've spent many years of your life engaged in full-time detective work just to find such an individual. Either that, or perhaps you've run into a rookie salesperson (who will undoubtedly be on unemployment very soon for being "too honest").

When you are selecting media, remember that the short-lived advertising you place in newspapers and on radio communicate a sense of urgency and "newsiness." These may be good selections if your message is about the latest surgical/diagnostic/treatment equipment, technique, or technology breakthrough, and if you're serious about running your message consistently for months at a time, and if you can afford the three or four times per day frequency that's often required to successfully "register" your message, *and* if you've developed a rotating series of single-themed announcements that have the right mix of creativity and visual or audio impact.

Limit the use of magazines to diagram and story-based presentations, and to long-term image-building. Keep in mind that magazine ads need to be planned well in advance. Most magazines require that your camera-ready advertising material be submitted at least a month or two prior to the month of the issue date desired. Magazine ads that coax readers into reading (vs. skimming or noting) are also most effective. Television (cable only of course, unless you're independently wealthy — *very* wealthy) gives the impression of "bigness," which is not usually something most doctors want to convey. Some doctors have used regional commercials successfully, however, when they're seeking to compete with area hospitals (ambulatory surgical units or walk-in emergency centers, for instance), or with large numbers of specialists in highly concentrated markets (to increase overall public exposure of a particular practice, for example).

Taken on a cost-per-person-reached basis, direct mail is far and away the most expensive medium available. The trade-off, however, is that no other medium is able to target the recipients of your message so effectively. It is said in major direct marketing company ranks, that direct mail allows you to reach left-handed, middle-aged, male college graduates with red hair who wear argyle socks on Thursdays. This is not to suggest that folks like that would necessarily make good Patients, but the point is that direct mail is a rifle shot compared to other media shotgun blasts.

Two words about direct marketing package deals that do "occupant" or zip code-targeted mailings of packs of coupons: Forget them! Save mailing programs like this for your cousin's auto body repair shop or beauty parlor. Professional practices stop being viewed as professional the minute advertising and promotional activity dips into the discount and special offer world. It's too bad more dentists, chiropractors, and podiatrists don't recognize this. Optometrists, on the other hand, like pharmacists, are not so negatively affected because they have come to be seen by many people as healthcare-related retailers, and it's acceptable for retailers to use coupons.

Reality Check: Unless you have a talent for conceptualizing and writing, and are genuinely interested in the dynamics of direct marketing, *and* are willing to devote substantial time to designing, testing, and delivering complete programs, direct marketing efforts are best left to the people who specialize in this delicate balance of art and science applications.

If you decide to hire a direct marketing consultant, check references thoroughly. Ask for specific results for each sample presented and judge the service on its attitude and general direct marketing experience (as opposed to experience with your particular specialty, which usually means very little). It's *how well* they've marketed that counts, not necessarily *what* they've marketed.

X

GIVING TALKSSSSSSSSSSSSSSSSS SSSSSSS (The 25 S's Rule)

Giving talks means getting patients. If you're not a good speaker/ presenter, or haven't made stand-up presentations in awhile, enroll yourself in a Dale Carnegie training program or take a speech course at the nearest college, community college or high school adult education program.

You don't like that idea? You're hesitant? Just the thought of standing up to talk in front of a group of people sends chills down your spine? It's okay. Don't worry. You're not alone. Research shows over 95% of us fear "speaking in front of others" more than other circumstances that represent genuine threats to life and limb. But this does not conveniently justify a policy of avoidance, nor does it serve to rationalize skipping over the next two paragraphs; it simply says you're not alone.

One doctor whose practice is fading, repeatedly denounces giving "talks" as "beneath" him and "unnecessary" because "...my grandfather, who was a doctor, never gave talks, and my father, who was a doctor, never gave talks, and they were both successful...." If it seems to you that giving talks is "too salesy" or "too commercial," you have an unrealistic view of the realistic needs of a growing practice in today's world. In addition, you are overlooking the psychic rewards that are an inherent part of teaching.

Don't make excuses about it. Do it. You simply can't afford to go one more week without taking a major step toward improving your presentation skills. In order to grow, your personality must drive your practice. How you come across when talking one-on-one is one thing; talking with a group is quite another.

If you are already a good speaker/presenter,
how's your "Talk Schedule?" (check one)

☐ A) I give too many talks
☐ B) I give just the right amount of talks
☐ C) I need to give more talks

If you checked A, B, or C, you need to give more talks. Simply put, good doctors can't give too many talks. If you think you're giving just the right amount of talks, you either don't understand the value of giving talks or you're not giving them the right way. When you give talks the right way, you'll look forward to giving them and, at that point, you should be generating a minimum of seven or eight new Patients per talk! Some doctors who work hard at this have reported bringing in 15 to 20 new Patients per talk with an audience of 50-100 people! Starting out with audiences of 15-20 and working slowly up to 30-50, and so on, is generally the most productive approach for building audience response and your own sense of self-confidence.

Selective Soliciting

Simply having "warm bodies" in attendance doesn't serve any purpose when you're speaking about a specialty. You need a select audience. When, for example, your target Patient population is senior citizens, your solicitation efforts must be channeled into the most productive potential senior audiences by the most effective means possible. This means you may want to consider setting up talks at nursing homes, depending on the age and physical needs of the residents, as well as the appropriateness of your specialty, and your own receptivity to Medicaid. How you feel about working with the older, less ambulatory segment of the senior population that nursing homes represent will also have a bearing on any decision you make to target this market segment.

Instead of, or in addition to, nursing homes, you may want to explore scheduling talks at senior residence homes and senior residence community areas, which now also include "assisted living" communities. Many resident and assisted living communities sport "clubhouse" facilities and activity schedules that include educational presentations.

Be sure to investigate speaker possibilities with senior citizen organization events and meetings, and with hospital-sponsored divisions, events, and programs that cater to seniors, e.g., information seminars focused on diabetes, cataracts and macular degeneration, arthritis and joint replacement, cancer and prostate problems, respiratory and sleeping problems, osteoporosis, vitamin deficiencies, Alzheimer's disease and memory loss problems, gum disease and implant dentistry, etc.

Start by designating an enthusiastic, organized staff member who has a good telephone personality, to phone target groups, businesses, and organizations with the goal of setting up "after hours" talks for you.

Have the same individual send a follow-up confirmation note and make a follow-up confirmation phone call to check on all arrangements, which should be neatly recorded on a large index card for your reference. Have the person involved develop an easy-to-read format, and edit his or her draft until it suits your purposes.

In addition to the date and start time of the presentation, and name and address of the group, notations should be included showing the exact location (which may be different than the group's address) with specific driving, parking, and walking directions (including a travel time estimate), number of people expected to attend, age range and descriptive profile of typical group members, total time allotted for presentation, if and when food and beverages are planned, and the name and phone number of the contact person. This card should be in your hands sufficiently ahead of time for you to review it before you actually depart for the session.

The individual doing this planning should also be responsible for securing, collating, organizing, packing, delivering, and distributing any printed and/or promotional handout materials, as well as any charts, pointers, slides, projectors, chalk, markers, posterboard, newsprint pad, blackboard, eraser, etc., that will precede, accompany, or follow your presentation. Finally, this person needs to send a personalized thank you note to the group from you the next work day after your presentation, with confirmation (or options offered) for a return engagement.

Be sure the individual doing scheduling and follow-up is guided by the need to make time work for you, not against you. Too many doctors have quit "the talk trail" because appointments were not planned with the doctor's life needs in mind (going straight from a full day of surgery or Patient visits to an out of the way location with no travel time built in and no time to eat or make a bathroom stop is a common example).

Smart Scheduling

The average attention span in our society is *12 minutes*. It can be even less with some age groups such as children, the elderly, or even other professionals (who often tend to be preoccupied, impatient listeners). Keep the time brief that you schedule for talking: 15 to 20 minute presentations work best, followed by 15 to 20 minute question and answer sessions. Be mindful of the groups' work or activity schedule and mealtime needs so you don't impose a presentation at a time when your audience will be tired or hungry.

In addition to the time of day, consider the day of the week. With less traffic than Monday and Friday weekend spill-over, and with Thursday being a major travel day for people taking long weekend vacations, Tuesdays and Wednesdays are generally among the best days for seniors to travel. Sunday afternoons are the best days for attracting other professionals. Monday, Tuesday, and Thursday nights are often used for club and organization meetings, etc. Also consider the week and month. Travel can be weather-treacherous and it gets dark earlier in some areas of the country at certain times of the year. Winter and summer vacation migrations as well as holidays and pre-holiday periods often preclude any kind of talk schedule. *Zero* attendance has been recorded by: a sports medicine physician who scheduled a talk for Little League coaches on a heavy game-scheduled weeknight; a (not sports-minded) urologist who sought to address a group of middle-aged men on Super Bowl Sunday; and by an OB/GYN who unknowingly set up a talk for mothers of pre-teens on a September night before the first day of school.

Regardless of how many people show up or don't show up, and how many are on time or not on time, *you* have a responsibility to be on time, every time, and to start on time, every time.

Showing Up On Time

Every doctor has to deal with emergencies, usually more so than other professionals, and the rest of the world understands this. Delay or absence at a scheduled talk due to a legitimate emergency is generally accepted and tolerated graciously when a sincere apology is offered and the situation carefully explained. But when there is no real emergency, there is no real excuse — *ever* — for keeping an audience waiting.

Plan your travel time so you don't have to rush, so you get to the intended location early (you can always sit in your car and read or do tape dictation or paperwork for a while if you're concerned about wasting time), and so that you can spend three or four minutes being a "detective" before you begin your talk. Use those minutes to get acquainted with the room, lighting, equipment, audience size, composition, and layout, and to thank the group's representative(s) responsible for arranging your presence. It's better to do "thank you's" up front in case you need to leave in a hurry. If you're not rushed at the end, another round of "thank you's" never hurt. Caution: Don't allow this important "prep time" to be consumed by idle chatter with the host(ess) or some other early arrival. Simply excuse yourself "to review some notes," then walk to the far side of the room, mumbling to yourself while studying a "talk outline" index card or two from your pocket or briefcase.

A gastroenterologist who must have thought he was some big-name celebrity rock star intentionally kept his first audience waiting for half an hour or so to "let them build up some energy." They left. He rationalized that they wouldn't have been worth his time anyway, and proceeded to repeat the scenario four more times before being rudely awakened to the fact that word of his thoughtlessness had found its way around town, and that no one wanted him as a speaker anymore. Needless to say, that reputation has not helped his practice. He's had to work day and night to try to turn around his negative image, and he may never fully succeed.

When you finally get yourself into the spotlight, remember your purpose and stay focused. It's easy to start trying to qualify for an Academy Award, or seeking recognition for your stand-up comedy routine. The best approach is to *keep it simple and speak succinctly.*

Speaking Succinctly

When someone asks what time it is, don't tell that person how to make a clock. Even some of the best prepared speakers who are able to give strong, interesting, crisp, concise presentations can have a tendency toward overkill when answering follow-up questions. Remind yourself that you are where you are because the group or organization already believes that you know what you're talking about and wants to learn. You don't need to try to impress them with how much you know. *Your real purpose is to have your audience feel they can relate to you, appreciate your authenticity, and trust you enough as a person to consider seeing you as a doctor.* Provide direct responses so that more people can ask more questions within the designated time period. Most importantly, *leave when your time is up, and leave people wanting more.*

Remember, the average education level of Americans is still reported to be at a point somewhere between sixth and eighth grade. Use short, simple, nontechnical words and give lots of examples. Storytelling is fine as long as it is brief and serves a specific informational purpose. Humor is fine as long as it's really funny (not just to you, your staff, and other doctors), in good taste (not just yours, your staff's, and that of other doctors), and appropriate to the audience (not just what you, your staff, and other doctors think is appropriate). Talk with the person(s) who make the arrangements for your presentation ahead of time to get a "profile" of the number and kinds of people who would be expected to attend so you can adjust/adapt your presentation to "fit" the audience.

Speak slowly, clearly, and with enough volume for the person farthest away in the room to hear you comfortably. Always speak in the same tone of voice and simplistic terms you would use in a private, one-on-one Patient conference. Take special care not to sound pedantic, condescending, or patronizing. People will know that you believe in yourself if you speak from your heart and sound sensible.

Sounding Sensible

A highly successful young surgeon has attributed much of his 50-60 Patients-per-day following to the boldness and frequency with which he asserts that he will *only* accept Patients and *only* recommend surgery in those instances where he is *very* confident of being able to help Patients get the results they want. He not only makes sure that all his printed materials emphasize this point, he goes to great lengths to underscore it as his standard policy every time he gives a talk (once a week).

To those people who believe surgery should only be used as a last resort, he sounds sensible. To those people who make elective surgery into an expensive hobby and always want "the latest" procedure, he sounds sensible. To those people who clearly need surgery, he sounds sensible. People think he sounds sensible. People like people who sound sensible. People *especially* like doctors who sound sensible.

Sounding sensible does not mean representing yourself as a mass of objective, unemotional logic. According to numerous current studies, articles, and books like Bill Moyers' *Healing And The Mind* (Doubleday, 1993, New York), even conservative, traditional, mainstream medical practitioners are beginning to acknowledge, and in many cases subscribe to, the existence and importance of psychoimmunology.

Psychoimmunology has been defined by former advertising executive and current free-lance writer A. Stanley Kramer in a guest-editorial for *Newsweek* (June 7, 1993) entitled, "A Prescription For Healing" as "the degree to which belief becomes biology — the interaction between the brain, the endocrine system and the immune system." The principle of psychoimmunology sets forth that your ability to communicate a sense of reassurance will be considered by many (perhaps the majority) of those you speak with, to be at least equal in importance to your clinical skills in their judgement of you as a doctor. So, "sounding sensible" with the presentations you make, to groups *and* individuals, means proactively embracing and verbalizing some positive attitudes. You need to project a posture of reassurance and calming influence. You need to demonstrate your ability to think and act rationally, without appearing overly serious.

You can convey a sense of confidence in your ability to help others feel more confident in themselves, and in their own abilities to use their minds to contribute to the healing process, by the way you handle your audience, particularly during question and answer exchanges. By doing this, you are not only helping people to feel a greater sense of hope about treatment and recovery, you are also "setting the stage" for attracting the kinds of upbeat attitude-endowed Patients you would like to have more of. Ask for and use audience questioners' names. This is especially important with radio call-in shows. It makes your answer and you, in the opinion of others, seem more personal and trustworthy.

One presentation vehicle that can help bring all of these "sounding sensible" attributes to the surface is the timely use of stories.

Sharing Stories

"Once upon a time," starts a dental implantologist's talk to a group of senior citizens, "a man named Charles Osborne contracted a case of hiccoughs. It lasted for 60 years. Between 1922 and 1982, he hiccoughed an estimated 430 million times. He was unable to find a cure, but, according to the *Guinness Book of World Records*, he led a reasonably normal life in which he had two wives and fathered eight children. Among Osborne's biggest upsets: he could not keep his false teeth in. Now, if he had seen me for a dental implant..."

Story Checklist

The story I want to tell as part of my next talk/group presentation

☐ **is appropriate for the specific group audience**
☐ **is in good taste and definitely will not offend the audience**

□ **is appropriate to the message I want to convey**
□ **is clear, short, simple, and to the point**
□ **is easy for me to tell without having to feel uncomfortable**
□ **will make for a more effective and provocative presentation**
□ **will help me to come off more positively than negatively**
□ **will fit the time, place, and occasion appropriately**

"Telling" stories is not the same as "sharing" stories, which requires group participation. Ask for audience involvement with the stories you tell. Invite answers and raised hands. Encourage note taking.

"Let me hear a good strong 'Yes' from all of you who agree that the kind of loud snoring I'm talking about can be upsetting to a whole family!" prompts a pulmonist of her audience. A dermatologist offers "I had a Patient once who was so bald he had to carry his dandruff around in his hand (pause for chuckles). How many of you have had a skin problem you've been worried about at some time? Let me see your hands...but not if they're full of dandruff! Let's count hands; raise them up high if you've ever worried about a skin problem." Of course everyone has probably worried about some skin problem at some time, but the point is that questions like this invite participation. People remember and respond to talks they participated in more than they do with those they've simply heard or attended.

Notice the use of "*How many* of you have had...?" vs. "*Who* has had...?" People are less reluctant to respond to an inventory or vote-type question when they are led to believe by your choice of words that they won't be the only ones raising their hands. Most people do not want to stand out in a crowd, especially if it's a gathering of strangers.

Don't hesitate to ask questioners to speak louder (or more slowly). Don't hesitate to rephrase questions you think others may not have heard. (Have you ever heard a speaker answer a question that you were unable to hear? How did you feel?) Don't hesitate to invite your audience to "give examples" when they ask questions, if you think that doing so will help clarify either the question or your answer. Don't hesitate to engage the example-givers in dialogue (especially when it seems someone is, consciously or unconsciously, attempting to "take over the floor"). In situations like this, be careful to show patience and interest without losing control of the presentation or the direction you intend it to go in.

When other people talk or interrupt, it's because they have a need to. If you cut them off or shut them down, you will be seen as disallowing their needs, and discounting them personally. You stand to be seen as intolerant, or even rude. You need to be seen, instead, as a little bit of sugar and a little bit of spice.

Sugar & Spice

If you have a natural tendency to be a bit spicy in your approach to teaching or conversation to begin with, don't get too neurotic about trying to be "yourself" or you'll end up with a completely watered-down, boring, dull talk.

If you are somewhat laid-back, sweet, gentle, and quiet in your demeanor, mannerisms, and tone of voice, stay that way. The only change you *might* want to work at may be to practice projecting your voice more, being especially conscious of raising the volume toward the *ends* of sentences (vs. the natural inclination to start a sentence clearly and then let the last few words trail off into a whispered state of oblivion).

Other than these kinds of minor adjustments, it's generally best to be your normally sweet or spicy self. And, as obvious as this may seem, it's worth noting that your success is critically tied to your ability to *know* your subject matter. You need to know your material well enough that you are able to stay alert to room conditions and audience responses and body language. You need to be able, mentally, to "take ongoing readings" of what's going on in the room so you can switch presentation gears when you detect interruptive outside noises or temperature or lighting changes — or the proverbial natives getting restless.

When you know your material "cold," you can deliver it smoothly and use your mind to monitor how you're coming across. Watch for signals of restlessness such as tapping fingers, empty or wandering stares, coughing and throat clearing, whispering or note passing, shuffling feet, people rubbing their eyes and faces, and people checking wall clocks or wristwatches. [If audience members start *listening* to their watches, by the way, you're in big trouble. Begin a prompt and graceful exit.]

When you detect these kinds of signals coming from more than one or two people, add some zing! Try getting more animated (or whispering) to make a key point. Try asking some "show of hands" questions. Try *anything* that departs from the flow you've established. [If nothing works, pretend people are listening to their watches, and follow the earlier instructions about a graceful exit.]

People watch your every move when you give a talk. Be sure to add a little sugar and spice to your body language too. Move about the room as freely as possible. Walking among the audience whenever possible is a good thing to do because the closer physical proximity keeps you in more intimate personal contact with them and helps hold their attention. Be sure to bend to eye contact level to answer questions from wheelchair-bound attendees. Refuse the use of a microphone (unless you're speaking in a stadium or coliseum) and a speaker's podium (which you would undoubtedly end up leaning on or over, like a lecturer, when people want to hear you "talk," not lecture). If you must use notes, confine them to one index card with key words and phrases (not sentences to read) to remind you of important points.

Be conscious of keeping that infamous "doctor's frown" off your face. Patients already think they see if all too frequently. You know that facial expression. It's the one that comes with the feeling of annoyance when you've answered one too many questions from neurotic knee-shakers who are convinced all doctors are out to kill them, or from smart-ass know-it-alls whose sole purpose is to try to trip you up in public. Just kill that expression right now. Standing in front of a group of people who are making judgements (regardless of whether they are conscious or unconscious) about you and your competency is not the place to show annoyance or impatience, or to chew up and spit out an interruptive member of the audience. More than one doctor has done this only to later discover that the interrupter they publicly devoured happened to be the group's "favorite son," key member, or major influence factor (the host organization chairperson's Alzheimer's-afflicted sister in one case!) And, frankly, even when the problem person is not a V.I.P., group dynamic studies show that speakers who berate, or react strongly to, upset audience members are not generally well-received or thought of.

Before or after your talk, some people may want to come up to meet you or make a personal comment to you. Don't leave any of these folks waiting — try to see everyone who has tried to see you. And, in these settings, be sure to squat or bend to eye contact level to answer questions from children or wheelchair-bound attendees. [Eye-contact-level communicating works wonders at bedside, too. Consider that one minute of seated or crouched position discussion with a Patient in bed is worth two minutes of you standing or hovering ominously over the Patient and/or the Patient's seated family.]

Selling Sizzle

When you buy a seat on an airplane, you're not buying the seat. In fact, you probably couldn't care less about how the seat is made or what kinds of cushioning, springs, framework, fabric, or stitching is involved. And you're certainly not thinking about the fact that what you're actually buying is simply the use of the seat, and the ability of the company that owns that seat to transport you somewhere in it. Why does this rationality rarely, if ever, occur to us? Because emotional buying motives always outweigh rational ones. What you are "buying" (mentally and emotionally) is the destination, or *the sizzle*.

Once in awhile, an airline will try advertising and selling comfortable seating, but never (except in targeting the small population of frequent flyers) for long. Most people who buy airplane tickets are actually buying images of places: Acapulco cliff-divers, historical Greek ruins, walking hand-in-hand with a lover through some deserted Caribbean surf, skiing in the Alps, family pursuits in amusement parks, pristine wilderness settings, native foods/music/costumes...the destination...the sizzle!

"Whoa! Sounds good, but I'm a doctor, not an airline. What does any of this have to do with me?" You're not an airline, but you do provide a service. Your Patients are your customers. Customer behavior, buying motives, and habits don't change because you are a doctor. Customers buy sizzle. Patients are customers.

Don't talk about mucosal blade inserts, phacoemulsification, chemical peels and dermabrasion, maxillofacial prosthodontics, and flexion/ distraction. Nobody understands all that and nobody cares. If you use too much clinical/technical language, you'll literally scare people away.

So, instead of discussing the types of inserts you might surgically implant into the gums, talk instead about the fact that the procedure will allow implant recipients to confidently bite into an apple or eat an ear of corn again, or how they'll never have to deal with the in's and out's of dentures again (the destination...the sizzle!). Instead of telling potential Patients about the instruments and methodology you use in doing cataract removal or hip replacement procedures (information you might share one-on-one in a pre-op conference), focus on expectations for resuming an active lifestyle and being able to see more of, or even lift, grandchildren (the destination...the sizzle!).

Chiropractors, for example, should talk about "guiding" the body "naturally" and making "gentle adjustments" instead of "cracking," "subluxations" and "scapulothoracic articulation." Whenever you're talking to "the outside world," *keep it simple*!

None of this is to suggest any avoidance of the responsibilities attached to "full disclosure" discussions with Patients. To not share with a Patient that she/he should expect pain, black and blue spots, inflexibility, nausea, or whatever, as part of a treatment or procedure, or its follow-up, is not only irresponsible, it will cost you severely in reputation, Patient referrals and, ultimately, revenues.

Probably the most important bit of *image*-sizzle you can "sell" (not just in talks, but in every day-to-day exchange) is to provide *every* audience you address (staff groups included) with a sincere sampling of the "real" you, the authentic you.

Don't be afraid to be genuine. It's really safe and okay that others get a taste of your "giving" personality (which you must have some of in order to be a doctor in the first place) vs. the stereotypical "taking" characteristics that many in the media and general public often associate with the superior income levels and lifestyles doctors maintain.

There is no better way to be seen by others than as a giver of genuine and deserved praise. When you take the opportunity (especially in your public appearances) to praise, or make "shining stars" out of those who work with and around you, you enhance your own image as well. The same dynamics occur when you can spotlight your audience.

Shining Stars

The best way to gain acceptance with any audience, regardless of size, composition, ages or affiliations, is to put the spotlight on them. Make those who are there to hear you speak into "shining stars." Point to your audiences' individual or group accomplishments. It would be unforgivable to address a Lion's Club meeting, for example, without referring to the organization's many contributions to the blind and visually impaired, or to ignore or not comment on the exceptional landscaping and grounds of the clubhouse where you're speaking.

Make sure, for instance, to call special attention to a particularly attractive brooch (or scarf) that the organization hostess (or lady in the front row) is wearing (assuming, of course, that you find the item to be attractive or "unique"). Mention an honor recently achieved by one or more of the members of the group that's featuring you. It obviously helps to do an initial workup on your host and host organization ahead of time.

When one member of a prominent internist group delivers a talk, he is always accompanied by two office staffers, dressed in their whites, who assist him with a short sound and slide presentation, and with distributing literature. After each talk, they actually book appointments. The doctor never fails to make a major event out of introducing the attending staff members. Each is given a 60-second "commercial" that praises the individual's strengths, attitude, devotion, understanding, popularity with Patients, and professional pursuits and accomplishments, and includes personal comments about their families or community involvements.

Corny? Perhaps, but audiences love it; it puts them at ease. The staff people involved may pretend to be embarrassed or uncomfortable, but public comments like this are appreciated. When what's said is more than just flattery, it becomes enormously reinforcing to an individual's sense of career commitment. And remember, sincerity is *critical*.

After such rave reviews, the audience sees each of these people as professional extensions of the doctor, rather than as strangers or "vultures hovering around the back of the room," as three unintroduced (whispering, no less!) nurse's aides were described by one couple attending an educational medical talk.

But the greatest benefit of publicly praising your people is that you increase your personal prestige every time you make someone else "the star of the show." Doctors who make "Shining Stars" of their Patients, staff members, and audiences, are those whose Patient-flow and revenue-flow "Stars" shine the brightest and longest, and actually become guiding lights for other professionals. [Some doctors use Patient News and Staff News bulletin boards to display news items crediting accomplishments of their Patients and support personnel. Staffers take turns skimming local papers at home each week, as part of their written job description, looking for any positive mention of any of the doctor's Patients or staff.]

While you're busy creating starlight with your left hand, remember to bring on some showers with your right.

*S*howering *S*ouvenirs

One characteristic of industrialized society we can all be 100% certain of is that everyone likes to get something for free. In fact, of the 450,000 "active" and 700,000 "dead" words in the English language, "free" has proven time and again to be the most powerful, most magical, highest impact word possible to use in any form of advertising. So, naturally, doctors can't use it, right? Doctors can't give away anything, they're told. Yet this is not entirely true. There are many "free" things doctors can legally and ethically give away, both in the office and at talks.

Remember Dr. Mack D'generayshun, the ophthalmologist who gives promotional tagged flowers to office visitors? He also gives them out at talks. The "Apple Dentist" gives out apples at talks. A sports physician hands out head and wrist sweat bands. Free information can be packed into recyclable plastic bags. Refrigerator magnets, especially anything out of the ordinary (in terms of size, shape, message, magnet strength, clip or slot features) are almost always well-received, kept, and displayed.

Where it's appropriate (and it almost always is), give the group or organization that's sponsoring your talk a Certificate of Appreciation or Certificate of Acknowledgement (Figure 10-1). Better yet, present a framed certificate. The best option would be to present an engraved plaque. Most of these kinds of items end up being prominently displayed. As such, they end up being "silent salesmen," representing your name in a positive light 365 days a year on a lobby or meeting room wall.

Promotional giveaways such as certificates, engraved plaques, and information packets must be planned ahead of time. Other aspects of successful talks need to be, or at least appear to be, spontaneous.

Spontaneous Scheduling and Rescheduling

Doctors who make the most of the opportunity to set up patient appointments "on the spot" are most often rewarded with Patient appointments. Attending staff people can do this very tastefully with your actual appointment book, or a copy, on their laps or at a table. Also, doctors who ask, "on the spot," to reschedule a follow-up talk even a year from the current date are usually rewarded with a prompt booking.

Asking for what you want works better than not asking. Asking for what you want works better than hinting at what you want, e.g., "Gee, it would be nice if I could return and talk with this group again some time" simply cannot be as effective or productive as, "Can we book a return engagement date for six months from today? Will the same time and place be okay?" Similarly, "Some doctors I know have been able to get referrals from this group for other talk arrangements" is nowhere near as results-oriented as, "I would greatly appreciate it if you would take a minute, right now, to jot down any organizations besides this one that you think might be interested in a similar presentation. Please include any name, address, and phone number you may know to facilitate the contact, and your own name if it's okay for me to use you as a reference."

The dynamics of asking for business-related arrangements differ from those you would use in asking for clinically-related arrangements. It's hardly plausible to imagine a surgeon in the middle of surgery *hinting* for a scalpel or clamp. In the O.R., for example, you may be captain of the ship; you command and you get. There's little room for courtesy on the

Figure 10-1

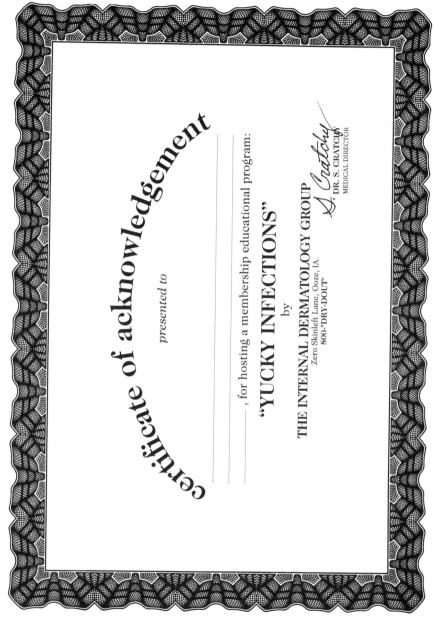

DECORATIVE BORDER © 1989 GRAPHIC PRODUCTS CORPORATION

firing line. But in business, no one responds favorably to a command. Asking for what you want means doing it with appreciation for the nature of the person, business, and environment involved.

Being assertive, asking for what you want, is not the same thing as being aggressive. Aggressiveness involves physical or mental/emotional harm. Language can be aggressive. The manner in which language is used can be aggressive. When verbal aggression is not directly abusive, it easily can be construed as rudeness. By contrast, being pleasantly assertive with your audiences can serve to communicate a sense of confidence and leadership, and sow the seeds of desire for people to want to trust you and your judgements.

Sowing Seeds

Stop being bashful, defensive, irritated, reluctant, or whatever it is that's been holding you back from giving vibrant, productive, meaningful talks. You're not lowering yourself to some despicable level. You're not "hawking your wares." You're not "slick-talking" or "hustling" people.

If you need an image to cling to, think of yourself as Johnny Appleseed, seeding your way through your community; scratching the surface, planting seeds, teaching the values of proper care. Realize that some trees will sprout and mature quickly, but most will need time and repeated attention. Above all, realize that you have important information to share, and when you do this in a manner that is simple, sincere, and straightforward, it will come back to you in the form of increased numbers of Patients and referrals. What goes around comes around.

Sweet Success

You'll find, rather quickly, that the key to "Sweet Success" for this whole business of giving talks has more to do with adhering to the basics of common sense, good manners, and clear communications than it does with giving a buttoned-up, carefully prepared and organized presentation of pathological indications and processes.

Year after year, we all watch professional teams and athletes literally stumble through command performance championships, after playing superbly all season, because they become so overwhelmed with the spotlights and clamor that they end up ignoring the basics. Stick to the basics. Be especially conscious of how you feel when you are in someone else's audience, and let that be your guide for how to present yourself.

XI

MAKING NEWS WITHOUT MAKING WAVES

Tenacity and the Squeaky Wheel

News releases are free (as opposed to advertisements). Stories that result from news releases are read, viewed, or heard with ten times the credibility of paid advertising. And doctors don't need to win a Nobel Prize, tightrope walk across Main Street, or rescue someone from a burning building in order to attract positive print or broadcast headlines. So why don't more doctors use news releases instead of advertisements?

Simple. Advertisements are easy. You buy the space. You fill the space. And you have almost total control over what you want to say in the space. News releases require you to play the news release game. First you have to write the release, but only in a certain way. Figure 11-1 shows an example of an acceptable format to follow for a news release. Next, you should package the release, but only in a certain way. Then, you need to distribute the release, also only in a certain way. After that, you must follow up *tenaciously* by phone, fax, mail, and — where possible — in person. Remember, "the squeaky wheel" really does "get the grease" when it comes to editorial decision-making.

Finally, you need to know that even after doing all these time-consuming things, you end up with zero control over what (if anything) is printed or broadcast because the editor or news director *always* retains total, subjective autonomy over what does and doesn't get reported.

Newspaper Columnists and Editors Remind Us:

- Odds are against news releases that have no news.
- What actually gets reported depends on many variables, including the strength and timing of other stories.

Figure 11-1.

Your Letterhead

N E W S for Immediate Release... N E W S for Immediate Release...

Contact: Name, title, and phone number of person to call with any questions about content of the release.

HEADLINE (Usual maximum is seven words; try to include practice or doctor's name)

Full date. Town/City/State of origin... Begin your release with the first paragraph answering the questions: Who? What? When? Where? If the editor or news director significantly cuts the release, odds are that at least all the pertinent information will be preserved in the first paragraph.

In subsequent paragraphs, focus on answering the question: How? At the top of the second page of the release: TWO OR THREE KEY WORDS FROM HEADLINE: Continued (Date)..Pg 2.

Elaborate on the facts, concentrating on the newsworthy value of your story and the appeal of your story to the community-at-large, as well as any special interest appeal to the particular audience of each individual publication or station you're sending the release to. The more personalized your release, the better the chance of it being used. Use positive quotes that reinforce the headline or main message of the release. Include statements from the doctor/practice director/practice manager/office staff/Patients/ Patient families, etc., *when appropriate*.

Always include a *clear* photo (preferably black and white) with releases to newspapers. Identify subject matter with a felt-tip pen, printed clearly on the backside of the photo. A paper that doesn't print the release *may* print your photo, especially if it's interesting or amusing, with a caption taken from your story, or one that you provide, taped to the edge of the photo.

Conclude by building in a reference about who to ask for and how to contact your office for additional information. This should appear at the end of the release text, and is in addition to the "Contact" information at the top of the release.

Always double space between lines and quadruple space between paragraphs. Always use one and one half pages maximum. To indicate the end of your release, use a bunch of these symbols:
    ##

- Even newsworthy material is trashed if it's buried in trite expressions, acronyms, and technical/clinical terms.
- Mistakes (spelling, grammar, facts) don't disqualify a release from consideration, but they do undermine its chances for being taken seriously. Accuracy is critical because the volume of material submitted (often, 12 to 18-inch high stacks of releases arrive every day) makes reporters and editors decide on your effort in just a few seconds.
- Don't exaggerate — it undermines your credibility as a professional when your release is filled with superlative adjectives. How much, reasonably, can any doctor be associated with words like "leading-edge, state-of-the-art, newest, best, most, latest, enhanced, unique, significant, powerful, ultra, innovative, advanced, greatest, etc.?" Like any overdose, hype kills.
- Distance is also a factor in any publication or station's sphere of interest. The Washington Post covers the world, but it isn't going to publish a story about a generous doctor's contributions to a LaCrosse, Wisconsin, youth group even though the paper receives the release and appreciates the doctor's involvement.
- Don't exhaust your imagination and pocketbook trying to stand out from the pack. Lime green and shocking pink paper leave journalists literally green and shocked. Elaborately produced (expensive) charts, graphs, envelopes,presentation folders and covers aren't worth the cost. Releases sent in bottles, tubes, tins, balloons, and gift boxes are immediately noticeable, immediately suspect, and never regarded seriously. Keep it simple.

Nothing helps in your quest to have your story told as much as repeated phone calls and personalized reminder notes to the editors, reporters, and news directors on your distribution list. Your messages, however, cannot be demanding; they must request consideration in a humble and genuinely sincere manner. This is one place where assertiveness usually backfires. On the other hand, it is a place where repetition sells. If your first and second and third release never make it to the airwaves or news pages, and what you are submitting is clear, simple, newsworthy, and follows the format shown, try a fourth and fifth time.

Editors like to see your news release "face" with some consistency so they know you're serious and not a passing, fly-by-night operation. An ongoing (monthly, for example) series of news releases will outperform one or two "quickies," which generally carry the implication of being overly self-serving to most news people.

Just so it's not lost in that last sentence, it's worthy of repeating a quick cautionary note to avoid wording that sounds too self-serving or conveys the image of "chest-beating." Similarly, do not expect a release that contains "broadside" attacks on anybody or anything to be seriously considered. Regardless of what you believe to be true, factual-sounding statements and opinions must be able to be readily substantiated.

"I'm gonna make ya famous, Doc." So sayeth the P.R. (public relations) expert who "already knows all the rules" of the news release game and wants you to retain his or her services. *Caveat emptor!* (Let the buyer beware!) You'll do better to work with your most creative staff person and deal with local media people personally, in a sincere and straightforward manner. They will tell you what you need to do to get their attention and consideration, and they may even offer you direct help.

Packaging The Release

After you're satisfied that you have the best page and a half, double-spaced, newsworthy release you're capable of putting together, then be sure it has been clearly and cleanly reproduced (it's straight on the page, enough toner in the copier, no smears or smudges, etc.). Remember the Editor's Rule of Thumb: If it's too much trouble to read, it's too much trouble to publish! Now you're ready to package it; here's a formula that works:

- **First:** Carefully highlight in yellow, or underline in red, the "NEWS For Immediate Release" line across the top. Do not use highlighting anywhere else; it too often reproduces as black on a machine copy, and many editors elect to work with a photocopy instead of marking up your original.

- **Second:** Paper clip (no staples) the two 8 1/2" x 11" pages together. Be sure page 2 is identified clearly at the top so it can survive intentional or unintentional separation from page 1 by the editorial staff.

- **Third:** Carefully fold the paper-clipped pages in thirds, "accordion" style, so your letterhead is the first thing seen as it's removed from the envelope.

- **Fourth:** Move the paper clip to fall just above the top fold, so that when the release is inserted into the envelope, the clip ends up in the bottom of the envelope to avoid being caught and torn by the post office cancellation meter.

- **Fifth:** Add any photo or supportive material to the back fold of the release (not under the paper clip, which can "dent" your photo and affect reproduction values) so that it gets lifted out of the envelope with the release and spills out from the fold when the release is opened to be read. Be sure whatever is included here is independently identified in case it gets separated from the release.

- **Sixth:** The envelope containing your news release should be stamped (commemorative is best) vs. metered. It should always be addressed to the Editor, Health Editor, Science Editor, Feature Editor, News Editor, or Business Editor, etc., by name and title. It's worth the trouble to call and inquire as to the editor's name prior to mailing each release. This step should be repeated every few months, as job turnover is frequent in large media organizations.

  Make sure you target your release to the most appropriate editor, based on: A) Media organization size (one editor may handle both health and science, for example, on a small paper); and B) The nature of the release. A doctor seeking start-up funding for a new medical business couldn't understand why there was no response to a venture capital solicitation-oriented release sent to health editors.

  It often helps to hand-print in red ink "DATED NEWS RELEASE ENCLOSED" or "DATED NEWS RELEASE AND CAPTIONED PHOTO ENCLOSED" on an angle above or to the left of the name and address on the envelope.

Distributing The Release

If you would like to see your news considered for appearance in a monthly publication, send it out one month prior to the month of the desired issue date. For a weekly paper, two weeks in advance of desired appearance is usually a safe bet. For a daily, one week is generally enough lead time. Be aware that Sunday editions of papers are often 70-90% printed a week in advance. Short of having some awfully hot news to report, don't count on showing up in a Sunday paper unless an appropriate section (such as new office openings, promotions, etc.) is traditionally part of these editions.

Broadcast media usually won't report "routine" kinds of news, such as office openings or promotions, but it never hurts to include news stations on your distribution list (leave out the photos). This lets the news stations know that you exist, and that you're a serious, public-savvy resource they may call for quotes on hot or feature news issues affecting the community or your area of specialization. [A podiatrist, internist, or ophthalmologist would make for interesting local television and radio interviews on National Diabetes Alert Day, for example.] Broadcast media also have a shorter lead time than print, and will sometimes even respond to a "same day" release if the topic relates to some larger, timely news issue.

The single most effective method of news release distribution is hand delivery. Some political campaign managers seeking to capture frequent, ongoing coverage of their candidates make a point of personally delivering their daily releases each night, physically propping them up on reporters' keyboards for early morning discovery. Periodic lunch, breakfast, or even coffee meetings with local news directors, reporters, and editors — even once or twice a year — can pay you back handsomely when the time comes for some wanted press coverage.

Following-Up The Release

The worst thing you can do when you've finished following the steps described here is to wipe your hands off and consider the task complete. Once you've done everything possible to create, edit, reproduce, package, and distribute a news release in the manner outlined, the real "news" is that you've only just begun.

You must resign yourself to the fact that you are going to pleasantly badger the people you've sent your release to, on a daily basis, until you receive acknowledgement that the release is worthy and will be printed, or that it's not worthy and will not be printed. In the second scenario, you'll want to find out exactly what it will take to make your release newsworthy, or what it will take to help ensure that the next time around, your efforts will be more likely to be rewarded.

What you're apt to find out in the process of gently bending arms is that the individual you sent the release to is no longer there, or never received it, or that the dog ate it, and you'll need to send or fax another. You may be told that more information is desired (this is a good sign; the door is open a crack), or that there's no interest in publishing anything this time, but to try again.

The seemingly empty suggestion to "try again" is also a good sign. Editors often will feel guilty at not printing or reporting something you've worked hard and sincerely and conscientiously to have considered, and they will make a point of giving you extra consideration on your next effort. Sometimes, they will also call you during the time in between releases for a quote on something; this can be even more valuable than getting your release printed because of the "expert" and "authority" images implied when you're cited as a story resource.

In attempting to follow up, you may run into unanswered phones and unanswered messages. Don't give up. Write a short, pleasant reminder note asking if whoever it is you're trying to reach has had a chance to review your release yet and offering to provide any additional information. And keep calling and keep leaving messages.

You may be told that the paper (or station) you're seeking coverage from will only run your release if you buy advertising space (or time) first. This, unfortunately, is the reality of many local media policies. If such is the case, either schedule some advertising or go elsewhere (or make such big news that you can't be ignored, overlooked, or bargained with).

Once you have "paid your dues" by plowing through all the news release game roadblocks, and doing it consistently over a steady period of time (12-18 months, for example, with a crisp new release each month), you will begin to develop a relationship with the local media people and will reach an acceptable level of credibility. At that point, getting their attention and having it translate into news coverage can become as simple as making an occasional phone call or visit.

XII

30 EXTRA DAYS PER YEAR (TO WORK OR PLAY) FOR $5000

Picture This

You have an extra month each year to do anything you want. How would you spend that time? What would you do? With whom? Here are a few ideas to get you started thinking (check one or more):

☐ Research
☐ Family Activities
☐ Travel (by) ☐ Car ☐ Plane ☐ Ship ☐ Other
☐ Spending Time at Home
☐ Reading
☐ Golf/Fishing/Boating/Tennis
☐ Yard work/Landscaping
☐ Workshop/Tinkering/Inventing
☐ Museums/Shows
☐ Build or strengthen personal/business/professional relationships

Now picture this: You can do 30 day's worth of whatever you checked off within the next twelve months for a one-time total approximate expenditure of $5000, and it doesn't matter what your specialty is or whether you've been in practice for five years or 25 years.

What's the catch? There is no catch. By following the approach outlined, you will end up saving three to ten minutes with every new Patient (or every pre- or post-op Patient, or every Patient with an ailment common to your specialty). Multiply the three to ten minutes saved by the number of daily Patients (20?) and you'll quickly arrive at a one to three-hour time savings every day. At five days a week, this translates to five to 15 hours per week, multiplied by 50 weeks equals 250 to 750 hours, or roughly 32.25 to 93.75 eight-hour days every year.

Getting Started

Write a five to ten minute script that you would use to introduce a new or prospective Patient to your practice or area of specialization. Approximately one-half to three-quarters of a typed page, double-spaced, will translate to a one-minute script, so roughly three and one-half to seven double-spaced pages should do it. Periodically time your *out-loud* reading of what you write as you go along. And *keep it simple.* The script could also be used for pre-op or post-op (or both) Patient (and family) instruction purposes, or for any routine Patient presentation in your practice.

What is this script for? You're going to record a short audiotape for new and/or prospective Patients. If you're worried that not all Patients will have cassette players, you can provide some $35 portable tape players on a short-term loan basis. If you think a videotape would be better, it wouldn't. How many informational videocassettes have people given you to bring home and watch that you actually brought home and watched?

The purpose of your script is to capture the standard three to ten minutes worth of "boiler plate" comments that you ordinarily rattle off and that Patients inevitably forget or digest more slowly than the speed with which you serve up the information. How often do they have to ask you to repeat yourself, or ask your staff people to repeat, or (after they've returned home) call your office back with questions? Your script is the one place to include all of your standard instructions, regardless of whether you currently use printed versions. Even people who can read rarely do. But everyone listens to the doctor.

The next step is to read your script draft over the phone to two or three nonlawyer, nonhealthcare-business friends. Professional speech writers try out their "wares" on taxi drivers, elevator operators, waitresses, grandmothers and children. Ask your listeners to pretend they are your Patients (or prospective Patients) and to critique the script for you to help ensure that it communicates your message clearly and pleasantly. Then ask your lawyer to review a copy (on a courtesy basis) *only* for any glaring potential legal concerns. Adjust the language as necessary. (The words "insure" and "ensure," for example, are not recommended in any description of treatment expectations.)

Production Tips

At this point, your total cost is $0, assuming that you haven't used revenue-productive Patient time to write, edit, and practice your presentation (and that you don't have a shark for a lawyer!). So when does money come into play? Beginning now. Once you're feeling comfortable with your script and your delivery, shop around for a recording studio. They can cost anywhere from $40-$240 per hour. Unless you're in a major urban area such as Manhattan, Los Angeles, Chicago, or Dallas, and you're planning an extravagant production number with Dan Rather introducing you and the Beach Boys playing in the background, a $40-per-hour facility will do just fine.

Local radio and television stations often will give you free recording and production time if you're already running commercials, or if they think you're a good prospect to run some. Either way, local stations will usually serve your purpose in the most affordable manner, but also represent a significant trade-off: engineering ability and creative assistance more often than not leave much to be desired. Local radio station production skills and experience are generally far inferior to what you'll find in private sound studios. If you have any doubts about the abilities of your local station, go straight to a professional sound studio for help.

Be prepared to spend at least one to two hours of studio time doing the actual recording, and one to three hours more for editing. How could a five to ten minute presentation take all that time to record and edit? Recording time includes time to set up microphone stands, time to determine best recording distances, whether a microphone muffler cover should be used (depending on how much you "pop your P's" and/or how "sharp" your voice is), time for you to get accustomed to using a headset, time to determine the best lighting and script stand placement, time to set up seating height, sound levels, master tapes, etc., and time for coaching you through some trial "takes," as well as the actual recording, rerecording, and playback time.

Don't get discouraged if a number of attempts are required to achieve the kind of sound, flow, pace, warmth, enunciation, and inflections that you are seeking. Even professional announcers rarely, if ever, get recordings exactly right on the first try, or "take." An experienced engineer will readily tell you that you're capable of doing better, and make specific suggestions about how to improve your delivery. Take advantage of the opportunity to learn from someone who spends a lifetime perfecting sound recordings.

A good studio engineer can also adjust the speed and "brightness" of your voice, and edit out of the tape most "er's," "ah's," and "um's," as well as pauses, side comments, coughs, self-deprecating cracks, curse words, and the like. For specific and appropriate emphasis, your recorded voice can be enhanced with various degrees of bass, treble, echoes, and reverberations, and can be made to sound slightly more personal, friendly, sincere, engaging, straightforward, and/or persuasive than you may actually be.

Original music or "stock" music (usable without permissions or scheduled payments) can be built into the opening, background, and/or conclusion of your recording. Properly mixed and edited, the use of music can help provide listening continuity, enhance the spoken presentation, audibly bridge, accentuate, and/or soften speaking voices or subject matter, make the entire presentation sound more professional, and generally make it more listener-friendly.

The bad news is that if you are not the composer or performer of the music, the price for any original music you use can be expensive, ranging from $500 upward. The good news is that original music gives you greater creative control, a specific audio identity, and some measure of exclusivity.

Your purchase of original music may entitle you to any number of possible uses, from exclusive rights in healthcare, to exclusive rights in your area of specialization, to exclusive rights in your geographic area, to exclusive rights for educational purposes, etc. What you get is what you negotiate.

To avoid having to wheel and deal, and to ensure total legal exclusivity in all eventualities, a straight "buy-out" arrangement is most desirable. When you buy original music outright, it's yours. You own it. There's no room for having to make royalty payments or having to argue as to who can and can't use it (like your biggest competitor or the local plumber or funeral home), and when it can or can't be used under different sets of circumstances (like when the moon is full, or only between midnight and 4 a.m.).

Stock music is usually free, assuming the studio has something available that's appropriate. Unless it's in the "stock," no copyright, or expired copyright category, or you have the appropriate written permissions, don't try to use existing music without expecting to pay for royalties, or be engaged in a lawsuit. Even the composers of the "Happy Birthday Song" must be paid for every recorded use!

Music can be used at the beginning and/or ending of your presentation and/or carried quietly throughout the tape "under" your voice. Music and sound effects must be used carefully and selectively. Improperly chosen, timed, balanced, or edited music and sound effects can ruin your entire presentation in a heartbeat.

A radio station will provide you with a master reel or cassette (ask for both if you're unsure what kind of reproduction service you'll be using), but will not run, or dub, any quantity of copies. A sound studio will provide dubbing service either in-house or via an affiliate tape-copying service. A couple of hundred high-quality, well-produced cassette copies, with printed labels, delivered in individual plastic boxes, can cost a few thousand dollars, depending on how plain or fancy you want the tape to be.

"Plain or fancy" refers to consideration of including a "J-card" insert (so called because, when viewed from the side, it's shaped like the letter "J" when it's folded) in the cassette box. This card might feature your professional profile, office phone and location (perhaps a map?), an outline of your services, even your photo in black and white, 2-color or 4-color, unless you're unapproachably convinced that this photo sort of thing should be reserved for rock or rap superstars. A J-card, as well as the cassette label, should show a copyright notice: "© Dr. Hy Pidermic, 1994. All Rights Reserved" is sufficient. Include any legal name that your practice uses, along with your logo and any "theme line" that appears on your other printed materials.

If you can afford a total investment in the vicinity of $5000, it's well worth the quality and peace of mind you'll receive by going to a professional sound studio and having their people make all the production arrangements. That way, once you've recorded the script, you do nothing else except take delivery of the finished cassettes (assuming routine production needs) two to three weeks later.

If you're new in practice, or have been through some recent financial drain that makes you *feel* like a start-up, and you have the creative writing and verbal presentation skills, plus the time and energy to do the work yourself with the help of a family or staff member, you can record the tape at a local radio station and make copies on a friend's high speed dubber (or buy your own for about $300). Cassettes can be purchased (lots of 100 minimum) from various suppliers (check local sound studios) along with individual plastic boxes, for approximately 32 cents per tape, and 20 cents per box.

You can purchase blank cassette labels in peel-and-stick form on sheets, and type them individually, or run them through a copy machine with a (perfectly-aligned) master sheet. Each label should show the title of the presentation (keep it simple!) along with your name, address, and phone number, the length of recording time, copyright notice, credit lines for any original music or announcer voice, and the names of the recording studio and engineer. Labels need to be precisely affixed to cassettes on the first attempt because they're difficult to remove once they're pressed to the plastic.

An important aside: Do *not* use an announcer or another person to deliver your personal message. The single greatest Patient value of this tape is the reassuring feeling each person will have that he or she is literally "Taking the doctor home."

Because Patients can stop and replay the tape and listen at their own convenience, there is very little need for repeating basic information and instructions. Follow-up questions from Patients, when there are any, are kept to a minimum.

And because the audiocassette format lends itself to being passed on to others (sometimes months or even years afterward), Patients will often share tapes with others, including their family members. Some doctors include special messages to the Patient's family explaining what can be expected of the Patient and what can be done to help. This is especially useful with teen, preteen, pediatric, geriatric, and nonambulatory Patients. A fringe benefit of this practice is that Patient friends and family members who are exposed to your tape, and favorably impressed with it, will feel they have "gotten to know you," and will often become Patients at a later time.

XIII

TIME IS MONEY,
BUT LIFE IS SHORT

"You get enough rest when you're dead."
— *Kevin Bousquet*
General Manager
Interlaken Inn Resort &
Conference Center
Lakeville, Connecticut

Since your grass always looks greener to others, you'll rarely find any
sympathy (except among doctors) for your ongoing battle with the burden
of uncommon personal problems and the relentless futility of hoping
every clock you look at will grant you a 25th hour in the day. After all,
time is money. This is important because you make more money than
most people. As such, you have bigger money problems than most
people, which usually means that you always have to be making more
than you've been making, a feat that is becoming increasingly difficult.

You may already be spending the equivalent of an entire month's
salary each year just to pay your insurance bills, for example. To
compound your money struggles even further, you become, in your
moments of madness, a prime target for bad business investments because
you are too often taken advantage of by disreputable and/or unqualified
financial advisors.

Spending 12-18 hours a day surrounded by pain and grief and
suffering and fear and upset and anger and depression and discontent and
denial and panic and hysteria and ignorance is hardly a mentally healthy
and emotionally sound work environment in which to cultivate great
gushes of positive energy for your personal life. But this is not a
problem.

It is an opportunity.

Remember that at least part of what drove you to become a doctor in
the first place had something to do with your love of a challenge. You

are achievement-oriented to begin with, so why shouldn't the part of your world that's most important to you, your personal life, warrant your most important attention and effort?

Don't dismiss this thinking arbitrarily because you happen to be a workaholic and have managed over time to convince yourself that your personal life and your doctoring life are one and the same. If you *choose* for them to be, then you must accept that this inseparability is a choice, and good luck and God speed to you. If, on the other hand, you really don't want to be so overwhelmed with doctoring that you literally have no quality time for your spouse or children or parents or neighbors or friends, then read on. As with your Patients, there is always hope for those who want.

When your home life is not what you would like it to be, stop forward motion! Take a few deep breaths and know that *you* have the power to make things change. *You* can reinstate or boost the levels of love, understanding, caring, communication, and cohesiveness in your personal life, as well as aspects of your relationships that perhaps you thought others should be responsible for (Chapter VI: "Scrub for Happiness"). You have the ability to create...

Harmony From Discord

How do you start to manage more effectively the relationships you are now mismanaging?

- *You start* by putting some basic awareness "on the front burner." You probably function more often from the left side of your brain than from the right, which means you are probably more objective, analytical, rational, and unemotional in your behavior patterns than most people. You are also likely to be more communicative, more assertive, and more outgoing than most. Put these strong personal qualities to work for you.

- *You start* by applying the same diagnostic and treatment protocol dynamics you use with Patients (the same treatment and protocol dynamics discussed earlier as an approach to make your practice healthier) to your personal life.

- *You start* by doing a "work-up" of your relationship problems, paying particular attention to identifying the strengths and weaknesses that you perceive to exist on both sides of each troubled relationship, and by determining what you think the "roadblocks" are that have been preventing the level of improvement and satisfaction you seek.

When you're dealing with your wife, husband, lover, partner, son, daughter, mother, father, and anyone else who's part of your innermost circle of life, you must realize that no one else thinks and feels exactly like you. You obviously know this to be true with Patients. With family and other "innermost" people, though, there's a tendency to believe that being of the same blood and genes automatically entitles you to assume you're all "of the same mind." False. No one among those in your innermost circle (unless he or she is a doctor, or maybe a successful entrepreneur or a big-city police officer!) is likely to have your sense of urgency, your need for immediate gratification, your analytical approach, your emotional makeup, your sex drive, your sense of self, etc. So stop acting and thinking like he/she/they do. They don't.

Develop some specific, flexible, realistic relationship development goals with due dates. Then design your immediate and long-term relationship treatment plan. By following this (workup/roadblock/goals/ treatment plan) line of reasoning, you can at least set the stage for resolving differences in a more rational manner than you probably have before.

What's missing here so far, of course, is emotion and interaction. But the overt presence of emotion and interaction during the initial stage of problem assessment never seems to produce feelings of mutual fulfillment or respect when relationship management is the issue. This is not to suggest that love and laughter, for instance, are counter-productive to a healthy relationship. That's almost unimaginable. What is suggested is simply that during the preliminary sorting out period, it's usually most productive to try to withhold both emotions and interaction and avoid further negative energy. Negative emotional energy is at the root of mismanaged relationships. Dissecting it logically, rationally, objectively, and unemotionally — without interaction — is just the beginning.

A food-for-thought question from a University of Pennsylvania student newspaper ad headline for a religious history program reads: "How do you get where you're going if you don't know where you're coming from?" As in trying to quit smoking with the use of behavior modification, you must first keep an accurate record of when you do smoke so that you know from whence you begin, or "where you're coming from." At this point of taking inventory, all the interaction in the world won't help to avoid putting a cigarette in your addicted mouth.

Is the suggestion here that mismanaged relationships may have something to do with being "addicted" to upsets? Of course. Those who must encounter and deal with such a complex array of other peoples' problems every day, can end up with a complex array of uncommon personal problems to deal with for themselves on a daily basis. In other words, you, as a doctor, can quite easily get caught up with and actually begin to *become* part of the network (or tangled web?) of problems you are confronted with each day.

And unless you are conscientiously committed to a disciplined, ongoing program or approach to stress relief, release, or management, odds are you are carrying around more than a few upsets in your brain, heart, neck, back, shoulders, gut, sciatica nerve, or wherever stress tends to lodge itself in your body, to the point of distress and disease (Chapter XV: "Dr. Burnout"). You are setting yourself up to *become* part of the problem.

When you deal extensively, for example, with depressing people and environments, you easily can start to unconsciously accept depression as a convenient and legitimate response to life. When this occurs, you may experience such depressed feelings *yourself* that you can literally become immobilized. Subliminal masochism? Perhaps, but whatever you call it, its official name is no more important than whether or not you had poor toilet-training as a child. So what? What matters is that you are aware that repeated exposure to upsets can be addictive, and that you do something productive about them. Like take a break. Or a vacation. Or start sorting through them by withholding judgement until you've explored the upset with an autopsy mind-set.

The high levels of interpersonal stress (punctuated by all the published accounts of disproportionately high numbers of doctor drug and alcohol addiction suicides) leave little room for relaxation or self-development. Doctors, therapists, counselors, nurses, healthcare managers, law enforcement officers, entrepreneurs, athletic coaches, and mothers have a tendency to find themselves in this situation more than most.

Doctors in particular have more cause than most to be acutely conscious of how frail the human body really is and how short the life each person leads. Yet this consciousness is seldom raised. How paradoxical that doctors — whose inherent purpose is to help people live their lives more fully — can be so unfulfilled themselves, too caught up in the day-to-day pressures of their own pursuits to enjoy their lives.

What percentage of your time is too busy to even pause long enough to appreciate the need to live each minute more fully for yourself? ____%

What are some ideas you have about how to change this? Jot them down here. Now. Really.

_____

_____

_____

_____

_____

_____

_____

_____

_____

_____

_____

_____

_____

_____

_____

_____

_____

_____

_____

_____

_____

_____

_____

_____

At what time today will you start to do one of the ideas you just wrote down? _____ a.m./p.m.

How refreshing it would be to simply switch gears and go home at the end of each day without having to bring a back-breaking load of responsibility along. But then there's that "it comes with the territory" expression wrapped like the caduceus snake around every daily interruption. Doctor lifestyles are invariably marked by a stringing together of one interruption after another, to the point where what is interruptive becomes indistinguishable from what is planned. "My life is one big interruption," notes a family practitioner, "but, you know, you just learn to actually plan to be interrupted! I have to rise to the occasion so much, that now I just stay up there," he says. "Privately, I like to think of myself as a wave-maker and wave-stopper...as one of the people who keep the rest of the people together along the way."

Like many lifestyle pursuits, the higher you go and the longer you fly, the easier it is to slip, run out of fuel, "confidence-crash," dissolve away into oblivious exhaustion, take the low road, say "screw it!" to self-sacrifice and social consciousness, set yourself up to be kicked in the ass one time too many, and rationalize yourself into thinking like a hermit and acting (even inside hospitals and group practices) like a one-man band.

Pearl of Wisdom: Hermits and one-man bands do not good partners make.

Today's healthcare revolution pathways call for you to encourage and empower Patients to become partners and active participants with you in the process of their own healing and preventive maintenance care (vs. being passive bystanders, relinquishing complete control to you). In the same fashion, you need to encourage those people in your innermost circle to work with you, to share responsibility for relationship mending and building. You need to do this with very gentle nudging, and by very consistent example.

For others to gain greater self-control and share in the responsibility for the feelings and behaviors sandwiched between you and them, you must be willing to let go of some of the control you've assumed and exercised. You must be free of hermit thinking and one-man band behaviors. Perhaps, you may even have to give up controls you've commandeered for a lifetime. These may be controls that you feel you are clearly entitled to exercise or controls you've stolen outright from others.

Keep focused on the notion that what you give up in control of a Patient, a Patient's disease, pain, suffering or well-being, you gain in

Patient respect for your examples of leadership, guidance, teamwork, partnership, and trust. You gain by what you empower in others, and in the accrual of more personal and professional authenticity — the stuff that ultimately (and in unmatchable fashion) stimulates increased Patient-flow and revenues.

Sometimes, Doctor, you will have to fight your way out from under the halo that others put *on you*, and fight your way off the pedestal that others put *you on*. It will be worth it.

The Doc Exchange

Some doctors purposefully omit the use of their "doctor" titles when they introduce themselves to Patients, especially in settings where it's already obvious (e.g., the examining room). There is no loss of respect, loss of face, loss of tradition, or loss of implied authority. When a doctor leaves his or her title on the door, desk nameplate, or pocket-pin, and introduces him or herself as Chris or Frank or Karen or Margaret (regardless of whether the Patient chooses to follow through and use the doctor title or not), the doctor gains credibility.

From a Patient's-eye-view, the doctor is quickly and quietly viewed as a real, down-to-earth, unpretentious, able-to-be-talked-with professional who is more concerned with fostering good one-on-one communications and helping the Patient than with preserving a sense of inflated self-importance, artificial authority, and unrealistic false controls. Allowing Patients to call you by name or title, as they choose, is the first step in breaking down barriers to Patient empowerment. *Patient empowerment, when everything else is said and done, is the future of all healthcare.*

Life is too short to worry about how important you think you are. Your true importance is determined only by the authenticity of your thoughts and behaviors.

Reality Check: Write your own statement on the lines below that best describes what you think "To thine own self be true" actually means:

_____

_____

_____

_____

Mark your calendar for six months from today to check back and read the statement you wrote on the lines above, and determine what may have caused you to change your thinking and feelings. You might be quite surprised to see what, if anything, changes — and how.

Just as six months can serve as a suggested transition period for self-expression, so can six minutes in other circumstances.

One doctor who didn't want his second marriage to go the way of his first, advocates a "6-Minute Plan" that he claims has proven invaluable for helping to keep his personal life in better balance. Every night on his way home, depending on the weather and how late it is, he stops off for "six minutes of intensive activity" at one of three "de-stressing zones:" the outdoor driving range for six minutes of slamming golf balls, or the indoor batting range for six minutes of hitting baseballs, or six minutes of video games at a nearby arcade. "Six minutes is just enough time to wind down and make the transition from the office, or the examining, treatment, or hospital room, to the kitchen, family room, dining room or bedroom (and) the other 1,434 minutes in the day go a whole lot smoother."

A useful two-way form of positive relationship management (with a six-week focus) involves the use of advance scheduling on a six-week wall (or refrigerator) calendar that the doctor's staff prepares, revises, and mails to the doctor's spouse once a month. The calendar displays all nonPatient-related appointments and travels, with room to block in family events.

Without some method for keeping track of what is planned, everything begins to appear to be *un*planned. That which is *un*planned can suddenly become the object of unfair complaints. "You share more at the office than you do at home!" "Your secretary has more to say about your life than I do!" "When are you going to pay as much attention to your family as you do to everyone else?" Sometimes such objections and angry attempts to suggest change by assigning guilt can set off a chain reaction of accelerated bickering and power clashes that ends with mistrust in a relationship.

Many of the sentiments represented by statements like those above can be short-circuited with cooperative planning efforts, like a six-week calendar, to set up and maintain a policy of accurately communicating the doctor's business and travel plans to the doctor's family, and the doctor's family's plans to the doctor. One doctor's office manager puts "sticky notes" to the doctor's wife on the doctor's briefcase before he leaves the office every night. That way, the family always gets travel and meeting appointment news on the same day that the arrangements are made. The actual notes are simply removed and "restuck" directly onto the family's master calendar. The doctor has served as messenger.

"It's awfully easy to take for granted the people who are closest to me when I'm focused on meeting new people each day," says a busy pediatrician. "I have to make a conscious effort to keep the importance of my own family in proper perspective." She reports that the combination of regularly scheduled weekly family meetings, spontaneous, quick huddle-style discussions "as we all rush through the kitchen and breakfast in the morning," and regular exchanges of work, travel, and social plans "helps a lot."

Having effective family communications can only come about when you've also established effective office communications. Any part of one communications system that's just one degree out of sync renders that system and all other connected systems, useless, and can only produce stress. Typical out-of-sync communications systems range from careless and improper telephone handling and listening skills, to inaccurate and illegibly written messages, to needlessly complicated and inappropriately programmed voice mail networks.

The Voicemailmonster

Pretend for a moment that you're experiencing serious stomach pain and instead of rushing to the local emergency room, you decide to call the nearest gastroenterologist. Your call connects and you hear the following:

> Thank you for calling Dr. Manny Belchez. If you're calling with questions about billing, please push 1 on your push-button phone now. If you're calling with questions about insurance or administration, please push 2 on your push-button phone now. If you're calling to arrange for a follow-up appointment, please push 3 on your push-button phone now. If you're calling to

confirm or cancel a previously scheduled appointment (and please be aware that cancellations must be made 24 hours in advance to avoid being billed for a cancellation fee), please push 4 on your push-button phone now. If you're calling to speak with someone in the business office, please push 5 on your push-button phone now. If you're calling to request a transfer of files or to speak with someone in the records department, please push 6 on your push-button phone now. If you're interested in hearing recorded information about Dr. Belchez's professional training and experience, please push 7 on your push-button phone now. If you're calling after office hours (which are from 7:30 a.m. to 11:45 a.m. and from 12:50 p.m. to 4:15 p.m. on Tuesdays and Thursdays, from 8:15 a.m. to 12:45 p.m. and from 1:30 p.m. to 5:50 p.m. on Mondays, Wednesdays, and Fridays, as well as evening hours from 6:15 p.m. to 8:05 p.m. on Thursdays), and you would like to leave a ten-second message, including the time and date of your call, please push 8 on your push-button phone now, and wait for the beep before you begin speaking. If you are calling to schedule an appointment, or if this is an emergency call, please push 9 on your push-button phone now, and then please wait for our announcement of medical services available through this office before you begin speaking. If you are not calling from a push-button phone, please stay on the line and our operator will be happy to assist you, or connect you directly with Dr. Belchez if he is available. Thank you again for calling the medical offices of Dr. Manny Belchez. Have a nice day!

What do you think the chances are that a Patient in discomfort will hang up and call a doctor whose phone is being answered by a real, live, attentive, compassionate person?

When Everything Means Nothing (Strolling Down Drug Boulevard)

All the greatest possible communications efforts, systems, and equipment in the world have no value whatsoever if you haven't learned that doing drugs, even "just a little," even with "careful monitoring," even though "(you're) a doctor and (you) know what (you're) doing," even if it's "just a bunch of beers" or "just a line or two on weekends," is simply *not* the way to keep up with the speed of the profession, to keep awake and alert, to keep going, or, conversely, to relax. It just *isn't*.

· If you have a real drug problem, you're not likely to be reading this. You know all of this. If you don't have a problem, it's likely you know of a doctor who does have a problem, who should be reading this. Can you step in and exercise some "tough love?" If you've had a problem in the past, you know that the warnings printed here, along with those that appear in thousands of books, articles, ads, and commercials are true. If you're on the verge, get off the verge. Now. Go see a doctor you have confidence in and ask for help. Today. Put down this book and call someone right now. Just say: "Hi, Doc, this is Doc. I'm on the verge of a problem. I need some help from you now. What's the quickest I can see you?"

While the subject is fresh, don't fail to pay some pointed attention to possible drug problems with your immediate, or hospital-assigned Staff (even, and maybe especially, with your most trusted associates).

Extend this same careful attention to your own family as well. In most cases, staff and family stress levels, as well as ease of access to drugs, is only a notch below your own. In some situations, they may actually be more stressed than you, and have even greater access to drugs. Periodic monitoring in the form of simple, close observation is generally sufficient. Stay alert, don't get hurt.

Staff Infection

On the subject of observing your staff closely from time to time, if whatever you see at your front desk produces anxiety or doubt, do something about it! If you haven't already, you need to reevaluate the importance rating of this position in your practice — it's a ten! It takes only one microscopically tiny slip-up by your front desk person to land you smack in the middle of a malpractice suit or state medical board or peer review organization hearing. Additionally, the extent of pleasant personality being exercised, in person and on the phone, will literally make or break your practice.

It's completely irrelevant how new or old or experienced the personnel are who manage your front desk. He/she/they must always be much more than just adequately or even appropriately trained. Your front desk person:

- is a triage expert *and* a super sales personality, *not* a minimum wage receptionist.

- is subjected to almost as much stress as you are, if the job is being done right.

- needs *continual* attention, reinforcement, training, and retraining. You need to think of this person as a capital investment in your practice, and as your personal "king-maker."

As soon as you stop thinking that these points are necessary truths, you run the serious risk of touching off an avalanche of stress for yourself, the rest of your staff and associates, your family, and, most assuredly, your Patients.

Life is too short to spend your time digging yourself out of holes you could have avoided falling into in the first place. The effort spent up front to prevent such mishaps will more than pay for itself with decreased risks, increased Patient referrals, and increased peace of mind — an important attribute of longer living and a happier, more productive life.

In November of 1993, an 87-year-old adventurer named Colonel Vaughn was preparing to set out on a 500-mile dogsled trek. The trip would take him to the starting point of a 10,000-foot climb up the South Pole mountain peak named after him by Admiral Richard Byrd when Vaughn was a member of Byrd's famous 1928 expedition team. The climb had been planned in celebration of Vaughn's 88th birthday, and when asked by a reporter if he was afraid of dying on his adventure, Vaughn replied, "The only death we die is the death we die every day by not living."

Another Self-Abusive Addiction

Because most medical schools either trivialize or outright ignore the subject of nutrition and nutritional values, it has become and increasingly embarrassing topic for the vast majority of doctors, who know next to nothing about what, when and how to eat. Indeed, doctors are often less informed than the Patients who come to them expecting to learn more. Accentuating this vast wasteland of knowledge is an absolute blizzard of poor eating habits practiced routinely by doctors.

Really now, you didn't expect the subject of this chapter to scoot past without some attention to your easiest-to-hide and easiest-to-laugh-off addiction, did you? You really must do something to improve your eating habits. Not just *what* you eat and *when* you eat, but *how* you eat as well. Enough of this vacuuming up junk food, swallowing candy bars whole, eating bacon and eggs over easy without silverware, and living on pizza, caffeine, and grease burgers for days on end. Enough. Enough.

Assuming your 26 swallowing muscles are functioning normally, and you're not yet a dysphagia candidate, the odds are your body is equipped to chew and swallow the same way as your local librarian, the same way as your mother, the same way as a rocket scientist. But you're using it in an abusive fashion. Did you ever watch somebody drive a car filled with cheap "sputter" fuel, or try to control a standard transmission car having no clue about how to use the clutch? The point is you need to stop doctoring long enough to eat more wholesome meals at a more reasonable pace.

Limit other activities while you eat. Kill the phone calls to and from your stockbroker, real estate/travel/insurance agents, publicist, investment counselor, accountant, and financial planner. Eat first. Chew. Digest. Call later. If you're not sure what fuel will best keep your body's engine humming along, find out. You need to stop abusing yourself. If you don't take care of you, nobody else will take care of you. If you don't take care of you, you won't be able to take care of anyone else. Doctors make lousy Patients. Time is money, but life is too short to not take care of yourself. Now.

I ♥ My Self

Of the more than 100 doctors consulted in the writing of this book, *all* of them acknowledged the fact that they could do more for themselves, and all expressed interest in learning more about improving personal relationships, particularly with loved ones. These two desires, in many ways, are one. In fact, it's awfully difficult to improve your relationships with others without first improving your relationship with yourself.

While there may not be any single magic answer as to how to keep your personal life together while being a doctor, there most definitely are infinite numbers of options. Each option is a choice. Each option shares the ingredients of common sense thinking, and Golden Rule-type, "Do unto others..." behaviors. *Don't brush lightly over this paragraph!* It's so simple, it will escape you unless you stop long enough to absorb and process how what is said here actually translates and applies to you in your present situation. You become what you think about.

Dr. Leo Buscaglia, in his book *Living, Loving & Learning* (Ballantine, New York, 1992), quotes author and self-help guru Leo Rosten:

In some way, however small and secret, each of us is a little mad.... Everyone is lonely at bottom and cries to be understood; but we can never entirely understand someone else, and each of us remains part stranger even to those who love us.... It is the weak who are cruel; gentleness is to be expected only from the strong.... Those who do not know fear are not really brave, for courage is the capacity to confront what can be imagined.... You can understand people better if you look at them — no matter how old or impressive they may be — as if they are children. For most of us never mature; we simply grow taller.... Happiness comes only when we push our brains and hearts to the farthest reaches of which we are capable.... The purpose of life is to matter — to count, to stand for something, to have it make some difference that we lived at all.

Family Cartography

This is not about group surgery with all your relatives. This is about a family map-making project to help you and yours get to that special place called togetherness. The process of getting there, the journey, is what it's all about, not the destination. But a "getting to" needs some endpoint definition to produce real feelings of appreciation for the progress, and fun, along the way.

Having the chance to sleep late, eat meals at a leisurely pace, and just put your feet up for awhile might be a perfectly fine way for you to spend a holiday, for which you might have done next to nothing in the way of planning. Most nondoctor people, though, including those in your family, get as much, if not more, enjoyment out of the planning process as from the event itself.

Growing together as a family or a couple is an ongoing process. Ongoing processes require ongoing planning. Establishing a specific, regular time (and "rain date") to hold a formal meeting with your family or partner. "The second Monday of each month, between dinner and bedtime, and if it has to be postponed for a legitimate emergency, it will be rescheduled for the same time on the following Sunday" allows a set time for the plans and activities for each 30-day period to be reviewed and discussed, and encourages higher levels of participation and cooperation. If emergency postponements become too routine a practice, consider holding meetings on a "first-chance-we-get" basis.

Use the meetings as an opportunity for everyone to report on progress and plans, discuss roadblocks, resolve differences, stay on course and make adjustments as necessary, and to reward and encourage. Keep the focus on positive ideas and directions. To help ensure success, serve as an example by withholding criticism and paying close attention to other speakers. Encourage note taking and feedback. Use an agenda (even art-markered on a piece of cardboard will do). Post the agenda a day or two early so others can see and prepare for what's planned, and perhaps add topics of their own ahead of time. Then stick to the agenda.

For *any* meeting, family, business, or otherwise, when someone strays from the agenda, lead the person back, gently. Express appreciation for the comment made, idea suggested, or concern raised. Explain that "there's only enough time available to deal with the items on the current agenda." You might want to note (agreeably) that the issue being raised warrants separate consideration, then perhaps suggest a time to follow up at a subsequent meeting. Next, direct attention back to the agenda. The items on the agenda must be the focus of the meeting, and must be dealt with first, before any new subjects are introduced.

Make a complete and wholehearted commitment to have these gatherings become a way of life, a part of the flow, something that is looked forward to. What's the payback? The meetings will work. They can even become spiritual events when you or others overextend yourself/themselves for the benefit of individual group members.

Personal development consultant, trainer, and author Brian Tracy offers a quote in one of his advanced cassette seminars that serves as an appropriate guiding thought for family map-making meetings and, obviously, many of life's other events: "*Every* situation is a *positive* situation when viewed as an opportunity for growth and self-mastery."

XIV

DOCTOR PARTNERSHIPS: COURTSHIP, MARRIAGE, SEPARATION, DIVORCE, AND PALIMONY

"Laaa-dieees and Gennn-tlemen: In this cor-ner, wearing the smile, white coat and stethoscope, weighing much too little...and just back from altogether too many hours of beating his brains in, I give you the one, the only...Solo Prac-titioner!"

"And in the opposite cor-ner, wearing the expensive business suit, the scowl, and the cellular phone, weighing much too much...and having just returned from his seventeenth meeting this week where he had his brains beat in by other people, I give you one of many...Group Part-ner!"

A Prognostic Primer

Once upon a time, you thought there was this magnificent glowing light at the end of your internship/residency tunnel. You could see it almost as clearly as the white light that you've heard such vivid reports of people experiencing at the moment of death.

You knew the light was filled with pride and prestige and the rewarding feelings that only a good healthcare provider could know and appreciate, that only someone who had graduated to the stature of "doctor" could possibly understand. And there was money. Lots of money to go along with all the good feelings.

You found yourself in the most enviable position of being wanted, sought after, wined and dined by prosperous, established group practices, or promising, hard-working new practices, or solid, secure, benefit package-based hospitals, or you stood to take that glamorous, exciting first step of hanging your own shingle outside your brand new solo practice.

Regardless of your choice, deep down inside, you knew that, at long last, your inhumanly exhausting endless days and nights of torturous struggling were about to end. You had paid your dues, and now it was time to begin collecting dividends.

Then you woke up.

Famous Partners

Laurel & Hardy
The Pointer Sisters
Laverne & Shirley
The Lone Ranger & Tonto
Gloria Estefan & The Miami Sound Machine
Roy Rogers & Dale Evans
Fred Astaire & Ginger Rodgers
Batman & Robin
The Green Hornet & Kato
Lewis & Clark
Minneapolis & St. Paul
The Three Musketeers
Crosby, Stills, Nash & Young
Cops & Robbers
Peter, Paul & Mary
Peas & Carrots
Dick & Jane
Frankie & Johnnie
Frankie & Annette
Mutt & Jeff
Rowan & Martin
Ozzie & Harriet
The Kingston Trio

The Dave Clark Five
Lucy & Desi
Tom & Jerry
Ben & Jerry
Three Blind Mice
Guns & Roses
Beavis & Butthead
Patience & Prudence
Moe, Larry & Curly
Thelma & Louise
Abbott & Costello
The Marx Brothers
Bonnie & Clyde
The Jackson Five
Bob & Carol & Ted & Alice
Ruth & Gehrig
The Dirty Dozen
Simon & Garfunkle
Fred & Ethel
Soap & Water
Bogey & Bacall
Dallas & Ft. Worth
Starsky & Hutch
Tarzan & Jane
Fire & Brimstone
Mickey & Minnie
Snow White & The Seven Dwarfs
Tom Sawyer & Huckleberry Finn
Cisco & Poncho

Burns & Allen
Cheech & Chong
The Allman Brothers
Salt & Pepper
Fat & Skinny
Cake & Ice Cream
Cagney & Lacey
Sweet & Sour
Jack & Jill
The '69 N.Y. Mets
The Crew Cuts
Cowboys & Indians
Coffee & Tea
Huntley & Brinkley
Amos & Andy
The Flying Wolendas
The Chicago Seven
Martha & The Vandellas
Gary Puckett & The Union Gap
The Magnificent Seven
Peanut Butter & Jelly
Burns & Allen
Butch Cassidy & The Sundance Kid
The Wright Brothers
The Mills Brothers
Oil & Vinegar
Reagan & Bush
Bill & Hillary

Circle the three partnerships that are most representative of *your* partnership experiences. Why did you pick these? Use a sentence, phrase, or key words to describe what you most closely associate from your past or present partnerships with each of the three you circled.

1)_____

_____

_____

_____

2)_____

_____

_____

3)_____

_____

_____

Think about what you have just written. Partnerships are funny things. They always sound warm and cozy and reassuring. They seem, to those without them, to be arenas of productivity. Yet rarely are they any of these things. Rarely do they work at all. And when, at last, one works, it almost never functions smoothly.

So, for the lack of feeling secure and self-confident, many doctors buy into working relationships with others who either share the same shortcomings, and thereby compound the problems each had alone, or they join with others who have such domineering personalities, they end up feeling like indentured servants. As those who are experienced observers of marriages (and especially those who have gone through a difficult divorce) will quickly tell you, some partnerships with one domineering person, and some with totally insecure partners, do work. But neither is healthy. And neither is likely to grow.

As with marriages, partnership problems are often exacerbated by hurried courtships. Many doctors spend more time and energy visiting hardware stores to shop for tools than they do deciding on a career team to join. As with marriages, partnership problems also are often exacerbated by awkward periods of adjustment that parallel a long string of strategically clumsy incidents, from premature ejaculation to fretting over who squeezed the toothpaste tube in the middle instead of from the bottom.

Partnership success depends on the ability and intent of each individual involved to make the most of many of the same principals involved in a successful marriage: patience, trust, sharing, tolerance, understanding, caring, communication, and teamwork. Doctor partnerships require more interpersonal involvement and commitment than the kinds of arms-distance arrangements typically associated with traditional business enterprises. If you're not well-versed in the use of these virtues and personal qualities and inspiring the use of them in others, or you're not prepared to emphasize them on a day-to-day basis, you're setting yourself up for an estranged relationship.

Maybe it's too late and you're already in a partnership that's not working, and you feel trapped. If this is the case, click to another channel in your brain. You're not trapped (even contractual traps are rarely air-tight), so stop feeling and believing that your situation is hopeless. What your situation may be, is logjammed. Logs can be moved. You just have to move them in a certain, careful way so you don't hurt your back.

Once you give up on a relationship, any relationship, you are saying, in essence, that either you believe you have no choice, or you have become convinced that moving or removing the logjammed logs is simply not worth it. Don't choose to believe you have no choice. Your "choice" is to attack a problematic relationship instead of allowing it to fester to the point where radical surgery is indicated. You can attack it the same way you would approach a Patient's problem. Be a detective. Observe behaviors both inside and outside the relationship. Do a lot of listening.

As you set out to dissect and analyze, keep in mind that emotions can be tricky to sort out and evaluate. Love, for example, is not the opposite of hate. On a continuum line of emotions, in fact, love and hate are quite close to one another. The opposite of love is indifference. If you were to look at this from a slightly different perspective, it might suggest that it's easier to work with someone who hates you than it is to work with someone who's indifferent toward you. Anyway, don't try to cruise control your way through whatever emotional factors may be involved. Acknowledging their existence is half the battle. Responding instead of reacting is the other half. Are you breathing?

Next, define the problem as specifically as possible. This,

incidentally, can sometimes be more difficult than determining the actual solution. Force yourself to write down your problem definition. Then edit it. Make it as clear and concise as you can. One very specific sentence is usually sufficient. Then, write your problem statement as a goal to be achieved.

Your problem statement might read as follows: "Crepe and Suzette are both good doctors, but the bickering that marks their marriage relationship when they're in the office together gets in the way of what I want for myself with them as a professional career-based partner relationship." Restate your problem as a goal or objective to be achieved by saying something like, "To influence Crepe and Suzette to reassess the ways their marriage relationship interferes with our professional practice relationship, and to help implement appropriate adjustments." Note that the use of the word "To" at the beginning of a goal statement helps put the goal in an active pursuit context.

Once you've written your problem statement, stand back from what you've written and begin to think of the most productive, most sensitive, most feasible, most realistic avenues you could take to reach your goal. Be open-minded and honest enough to consider the possibility that *you* might be more of a problem than the people your problem statements target.

After you've determined these "avenues" (or *strategies*), write them down. Use action words to start each one, such as "*Talk* directly with Crepe and Suzette." Finally, write down the actual steps (or *tactics*) you will take to implement the strategies to reach the objective(s). This is the "do it" part: "Invite Crepe and Suzette to dinner (*or dessert!*) Saturday night and introduce the problem as part of a general update or practice overview discussion. Keep focused on specific behaviors that will help cultivate and maintain stronger professional work relationships. Solicit input and feedback about specific things I can do to help."

Partnerships are not always all they're cracked up to be. "Safety in numbers" depends on who's counting. It matters not whether you are a private practice seeking to join a group or add a partner, a group seeking to add a private practice or partner, or whether you are on a shopping trip to become part of an HMO, PPO, EPO, IPA, or a formal or informal network or hospital-based practice. Be direct and to-the-point in your communications with prospects. Figure 14-1 provides a solid outline for negotiating your way into a professional relationship.

Even after a totally agreeable relationship has been negotiated, the dynamics of a new partner entering a practice can quickly undo all of the

Figure 14-1

When You're Negotiating

1. Responsibility for a successful relationship is 50/50. Both sides must recognize and acknowledge this before any negotiations can be useful.

2. A Contract has to be entered freely. Agreements made under coercion don't last. If people haven't freely chosen to agree, they're not ready for a contract.

3. There must be consideration from both sides. You can't get something for nothing, even in a senior partner/junior partner or practice director/staff doctor relationship.

4. All wants are legitimate. People want what they want and are entitled, by birth, to express those wants.

5. You don't always get what you want. And that's ok.

6. You can say no. This applies even in boss/subordinate relationships. Saying that you can't say no really means you don't want to deal with the consequences of saying no. [If the consequences mean no job and you can't afford that, you must respond from your sense of integrity, or be prepared to live with long-term guilt or a short-term lesser job.]

7. You can contract only for behavior and results. It's useless to try to contract for attitudes or emotions (e.g., loyalty, enthusiasm, empathy). People can't change their feelings; they can change their behavior.

8. You can't ask for something the other person or entity doesn't have. Nor can you promise something you don't have.

9. You can't contract with people who are not in the room.

10. Put the agreement in writing. This is the best way to make sure both parties are agreeing to the same thing. Usually two meetings, with the writing done in between, are required.

11. Include contingency plans. If Dr. A. doesn't deliver, what will Dr. A. and Dr. B. do? This creates a way for the agreement to last through change and/or violation.

12. Include some provisions for measuring progress.

Reprinted with permission from *Managing Differences & Agreement* by C. James Maselko, Designed Learning, Inc., Plainfield, NJ, 1985.

---

good intentions of everyone involved. It is imperative that sufficient preparation (introductory meetings, an on-the-job trial period if possible, circulation of resume/CV/biographical data, announcement cards/letters/ads/news releases, etc.) has been done to help associates, staff, and Patients accept the new person's background training and experience, face, stature, age, philosophy, attitude, personality, approach, family, and personal interests.

A new associate should have the opportunity to meet and get acquainted with every single person in an organization before actually starting work. There's no such thing as a second first impression. It makes no difference, by the way, if the staff numbers two or two hundred. Those who clean the office at night should be included equally with those who share in diagnosis and treatment protocol. Why? Because change, especially when it's done to people (vs. when they participate in the decision-making), can seem literally life-threatening. It thus becomes critically important to ensure that everything possible is done to help smooth the way for both the new person and the existing staff. This could take months of personal, in-office introductions to returning Patients. Each introduction must be as sincere and enthusiastic as those made on the very first day.

Calling It Splits

It's a fact that some partnerships end in separation and divorce. When this occurs, it is essential to "call it splits," vs. "calling it quits." Doctoring is a small world. The combination of the "insider" clubhouse ambience fostered by training and titles, along with the advent of professional networking and the rapid growth of telecommunications over the past few years has caused doctoring to become a very small world indeed. Doctors who don't know one another can quickly change that just by asking. It's been theorized that any intelligent person should be able to communicate directly with anyone else in the world by making three phones calls or less. If doctoring in those terms can be considered "small world," then negative relationships — bad blood, ill feelings, conflict, and burned bridges — make it smaller yet.

Unlike lawyers, who are necessarily adversarial by nature (because they never know what "fellow lawyer" they may face in court the next day), you, as a doctor, have an inherent consultative camaraderie underpinning your profession.

No matter how much you may dislike another doctor, it's never worth having other doctors know your true feelings. In a split partnership, it's best to smile, take a deep breath, and walk away, leaving the other person convinced you have appreciated the experience and opportunity to work together, and plan to remain friends.

If this seems to run counter to previously expressed ideas about being direct and assertive, it's because partner-splitting calls for a distinct set of diplomatic skills. The reason for this is that even though you are no longer going to be living (or working) with the person involved, you are going to remain within living (or working) distance. And what about potential referrals? Even if one of you moves far away, doctoring remains a small world, and continues to shrink with every consult, fax, teleconference, and satellite transmission. With every new drug, technique, and piece of equipment, often with the news coverage alone of journal article findings and reports, you are finding yourself working more "closely" with your fellow doctors.

On the subject of "palimony," trial periods are very much in order for any kind of doctor partnerships. Law suits for lack of trial period performance are not. Bonus arrangements based on trial period performance are fine. Fines are not fine. If it takes negative reinforcement to stimulate performance, it's time to change partners or partnership prospects — on the spot.

When you make up your mind that a partnership, personal or professional, is going to work, acting sincerely toward that end on a daily, even hourly, basis increases the odds of success probably a thousandfold. You don't need to plan extensively for the possibility of splitting up, but it definitely makes good sense to be aware of that possibility and your options. Be prepared to deal positively with any negative energy and emotions that might arise.

XV

DR. BURNOUT

You've heard all the stories: scalpels flung in rage into O.R. doors; clamps and hypodermic needles waved menacingly in nurses' faces; pages torn from Patient charts and ripped to shreds; Patient chart clipboards smashed over bed rails or uplifted knees, or flung angrily down the hallway or through a window.

You know all the symptoms: short fuse; impatience; the jitters; too much caffeine; too many cigarettes and/or alcoholic drinks and/or drugs; temper tantrums; increased volume of voice; less attention to personal hygiene and dress; increased fatigue; increased frequency and number of errors; less attention to health and fitness; increased tendency toward infection, muscle aches and pains, depression, lack of concentration, etc.

Like a parade heading down the street, you can see it coming; and the grand marshal, returning from Chapter III where it is credited with breeding ineffective delegation, is none other than good old compulsiveness, now breeding a form of death-by-doctoring.

Compulsiveness Breeds Burnout

Stop thinking you are the only one who can do things right. You may very well be the only one who can do things your way, but who says your way is the right way, or the best way, or the only way? You need to be able to delegate, then let go. Successful delegating is not so much a matter of the extent to which you trust others as it is a matter of how much you trust yourself, and your own judgement.

On a scale from 1-10 (10 = most), how much do you trust yourself? ____

The act of delegation should be no more difficult than the act of prescription. Someone needs a pain killer or heat applications, you prescribe a pain killer or heat applications. You need work load relief, you delegate some of the work load. Note that effective, day-to-day delegation usually involves a request instead of a command (ask, don't tell). To help ensure cooperation, limit your *order*-giving to emergencies, surgery, and complex or risky diagnostic or treatment procedures.

The 1993 World Series featured a Philadelphia Phillies starting pitcher who repeatedly reduced himself to covering his head with a towel to avoid having to watch the team's (high-speed but often reckless-throwing) star relief pitcher each time he came into a game to take over in a tense situation. You may have to cover your eyes the first time or two that you ask someone else to do a task that you always have done yourself. And sometimes it's okay not to watch. It's not okay to ignore or avoid the first delegated effort. Constructive adjustments can be made only when you're aware of an action occurring or a particular method being used. Just be sure your feedback is: A) Necessary, B) Constructive, and C) Reassuring.

Unless your practice emphasizes an assembly-line mentality, *how* a task is done is usually less important than the fact that it gets done. Of course this question of methodology choices has to do with waiting room magazine arrangements and scheduling detail rep calls, not with medication preparation or administration, or with adherence to board certification restrictions and responsibilities.

When you are afraid to let go, to delegate and walk away, stop yourself. Take a deep breath. Then, once again (as is suggested in Chapter III), rely on the answer to that all-important, call-to-reality question: What's the worst thing that can happen? If the answer is that poor performance of a delegated task won't destroy your practice or reputation, and won't hurt or alienate other Staff people or Patients or Patient families, it's probably safe to proceed without worrying.

Compulsiveness rears it's ugly head in other ways. Chances are good that if your behavior is the least bit compulsive, you probably are also working what most people would consider to be intolerably long hours. You may even have tried to convince yourself that you actually enjoy it. You may even *believe* that you actually enjoy it, but odds are that your work indulgences are simply excuses for not facing up to family life demands or upsets, or to other personal attention needs.

Excessive work hours on an ongoing basis often can be an unconscious protective barrier used to prevent others from getting close. It's hard to justify or set aside social time, for instance, when you constantly have to deal with your work load. Work becomes a convenient way to excuse yourself, a convenient way to gain the sympathy and concern of others, and a convenient way to think you have positioned yourself on the doorstep of martyrdom.

Workload Assessment Questions

If you are working an excessive number of hours, take a break long enough to *honestly* evaluate whether you're keeping the schedule you currently have because A) you really want to, B) you really need to, or C) you set yourself up to fulfill the expectations of others. Is it: A)? B)? C)? (circle one).

Hint: There's only one honest answer.

What are your three most important nonwork-related issues that need to be addressed or confronted, that you've been avoiding or putting off continually? Write them below:

1. _____

2. _____

3. _____

Are you using your work load as a roadblock?

If there's even the slightest indication that you are overworking yourself to impress or please others, or to confirm the image you think others have of you as "hardworking" (which you have somehow come to equate with desirable life virtues and qualities), you are probably deluding yourself. You have quite likely painted yourself into a corner on this issue. Your behavior, all by itself, may be perpetuating the myth that "hardworking" is a wonderful trait to have ascribed to yourself. It isn't.

"Smartworking" is a wonderful trait to have ascribed to yourself. Smartworking includes (importantly) skillful delegation. Skillful delegation demands skillful approaches to negotiating. Skillful negotiating — the kind that generates feelings of empowerment and longer-lasting, more meaningful results — requires a win-win attitude. Win-win attitudes start by sitting (both literally and figuratively) on the same side of the table as the party you're negotiating with.

The other party needs to get the message clearly that you consider him or her a teammate and that you're going to focus on issues, actions, behaviors, and things, as opposed to individuals, opinions, and personalities. You need to convey the message that you're going to work out problems, arrange delegation priorities, plan strategy, and relate to one another in a cooperative shoulder-to-shoulder manner instead of a confrontational, face-to-face manner.

How you respond to others' reactions will largely determine the level of confidence that others place in you. High confidence levels among associates and Staff help minimize negative conflict.

"A spoonful of truth helps the tantrums go down," is the philosophy of one softly smiling head O.R. nurse. Moments earlier she defused a potentially major conflict by very calmly and carefully paraphrasing the surgeon's screamed instructions to throw the surgical instrument tray "out the damn window!" In her honest, objective, rational, unemotional, adult-like, and gently humorous response to the temper tantrum-throwing surgeon's tirade, she quietly asked: "Do I understand you correctly, Doctor, that you want me to take this entire tray of sterilized instruments through these electronic doors behind me, down the hall to the window, open the window, and throw it out the window, right now, while you're working inside this patient's stomach?"

Even the doctor had to smile. Calm was restored. The incident lasted but an instant. The operation was a success. In the end, the doctor was grateful. Of course the slightest vocal intonation or suggestion of sarcasm in the nurse's question could have triggered a disastrous reaction by the doctor. So, once again, it's the *way* that information is communicated or responded to that spells the difference between success and failure in an emotionally-charged setting. Under the circumstances, any doctor who would be *further* provoked probably needs professional help and shouldn't be in the O.R. to begin with.

Surprising as it may seem to some, conflict management does not mean that you need a black belt around your waist, a bulletproof vest under your lab coat, and a canister of mace hanging from your key ring. It does mean that you need to pay particularly careful attention to every word and emphasis you use at times when conflict may be staring you in the face, or looming ominously on the horizon.

Reputable conflict management training programs point repeatedly to the importance of using the words, "How?" when you're tempted to ask "Why?" and "And" when you're tempted to use "But." "But why?" you may ask. Think about this question. "But" sets up an argumentative posture. "Why?" gets you nowhere on the progress charts. What is the only kind of answer possible when you ask a "Why?" question? Imagine the response to any of these questions:

? "*Why* were you late this morning?" (Do you think there's a possibility the answer might have something to do with traffic or car problems? A broken alarm clock, shoelace, button, or zipper? Not feeling well? Not sleeping well? Not eating well? A family problem? A dog or cat problem? *Do any of these answers serve any purpose toward preventing future lateness?*)

? "*Why* is Mr. Todd's chart missing?" (Might you hear back that someone must have taken it, moved it, or eaten it? That maybe it's filed under "Mr.," by mistake? that a CIA, FBI, IRS, MBE, PRO or HIP-HOP agent purchased it for cash? *Do any of these answers help prevent future chart misplacements?*)

? "*Why* did you tell Dr. Bacbuster she shouldn't see our two spine cases until I change their prescriptions?" ("Because I thought you said..." or "Well, the reason is that remember the other day when you told Dr. Bacbuster that you wanted her to..." could be typical responses. *Do either of these types of answers prevent or minimize the chance of future miscommunication?*)

? "*Why* did you tell Mrs. Abbey to stop taking her vitamins?" (A likely answer might be, "Well, I know you don't believe in vitamins..." or "I wasn't sure if they would react to the pills you gave her so..." or "My friend never got anything out of that brand, and..." *Do any of these answers prevent future misdirections?*)

? "*Why* did you say 'an enema a day keeps the doctor away' to Mr. Katzev?" (Might possible responses include things like, "Mr. Katzev likes to kid around. I wasn't serious even though I might have sounded that way," or "When he told me he feels clogged up, I didn't know he meant in his nose..." *Do any of these answers prevent future misconceptions?*)

? "*Why* did you send Mrs. Megafuss' daughter to the pediatrician before I had the chance to see her?" ("You were so busy, doctor, and it seemed like the girl just had a basic chest pain/stomach ache type of flu..." or "From the paperwork the mother filled out, it sounded to me like a specialist should...")

"*Why ask why?*" asks a popular advertising campaign. Why, indeed? If you read the statements above, you can begin to see that every single time a "Why?" question is asked, the automatic response triggered is a reason, an excuse. And nothing productive can come of it because the excuse will only trigger additional upsets, and eventually escalate into full-blown conflict. What's the solution? Start using "How?" as in the following examples:

✓ "*How* can you avoid being late again?" (Effectively followed with a request for a list of specific ways to avoid being late, to review by the end of the day.)

✓ "*How* will we prevent charts (like Mr. Todd's) from being misplaced in the future?" (Follow up with, "I'd like you to please review our existing policies about handling Patient charts, and prepare a list of recommendations we can review by the end of the day that suggests ways to tighten these policies.")

✓ "*How* can we make sure that communications with other doctors (like the situation with Dr. Bacbuster) never include opinions or assumptions of anyone other than myself?" (Follow up with, "Please give this some thought and let me know by lunchtime what specific steps you think we should take.")

✓ "*How* can I communicate more clearly with you the importance of not offering advice to Patients (as with Mrs. Abbey) no matter how knowledgeable you may be about the issue at hand?" (Follow-up: "I will appreciate it if you will give me a list of learning methods that are most effective for you, such as one-on-one talks, memos, cassette recordings, etc., by tomorrow morning, so that I can feel reassured that the information I am communicating to you is being absorbed.")

✓ "*How* can you make sure that what you say to a Patient (like when you thought you were kidding with Mr. Katzev) won't be taken the wrong way, or worse, set me up for a lawsuit or Board inquiry?" (Follow-up: "Please give me a written statement I can take home tonight that explains what you think will be the best way to ensure that Patients don't get the wrong ideas from comments made with cheerful intent, without losing your sense of cheerfulness.")

✓ "*How* can we make sure that Patients (like Mrs. Megafuss' daughter) are not sent to another doctor before I've had a chance to see them?" (Follow-up: "I would like you to please outline a policy statement about this that I can review first thing in the morning, and that we can print up for other and/or new staff people to be aware of. Include specific steps to follow for referring a Patient elsewhere.")

Notice in each instance, the emphasis is on *how* to do something productive that helps to avoid or prevent the same problem from recurring in the future (vs. the typical reactionary approach, which is to dwell on the error and try to place blame or "nail" the individual involved). Dwelling on errors and seeking to place blame achieves nothing except alienation, disrespect, fear, cringing, and emotional outbursts. When you spotlight negative behavior, you beget more negative behavior. And, worst of all, the negative behavior becomes contagious. Also, in each case, the focus on *how* is underscored with the inclusion of a deadline (i.e., "by the end of the day," "by lunchtime," "by tomorrow morning"), and a pointed request for specific information. In this way, action is prompted (better than no action, remember?) rather than run the escalating risks associated with delays.

Notice also, that the burden of responsibility for solving the problem is turned over to the person whose behavior is the source of the problem. When you accept responsibility for solving other peoples' problems, you set yourself up for a lifetime of problem-solving for those individuals.

With the "How?" approach, the emphasis is on a behavior or policy or procedure, rather than on the person or personality of the individual involved. The attack is on Sally's behavior, not on Sally as a person. The result is defused emotions, undamaged egos, and a markedly increased potential for creating forward movement out of a backward step.

Such are the subtleties of shifting emphasis brought on by changing a single word. Similarly, the prospects for engaging conflict are substantially reduced (often, in fact, reversed) by conscious use of the word "and" in place of "but," as with these examples:

• "I agree with your thinking that we need to decrease receivables, *but* I think the responsibility for making that happen rests with the office staff" is not as effective as "I agree with your thinking that we need to decrease receivables, *and* I think the responsibility for making that happen rests with the office staff."

• "You certainly are correct in identifying appointment scheduling as a growing problem for our Patients, *but* this is an area for you to exercise your responsibilities" is not as effective as "You certainly are correct in identifying appointment scheduling as a growing problem for our Patients, *and* this is an area for you to exercise your responsibilities."

Another important anti-conflict tactic worth noting that surfaces in these comparisons is that the other person's point of view is first supported ("I agree with your thinking that...") before being confronted. When "but" is used to set up the confrontational part of the statement, it tends to discredit the opening, supportive comment. On the other hand, when "and" is substituted for "but," it tends to enhance the supportive comment. Caution: "however" and "though" are simply other ways of saying "but," and are subject to the same negative thinking and dynamics expressed for "but."

How To Deal With Anger

When someone is yelling in your face, the situation requires immediate action. There's no time to start sorting out whether to use "why" or "how" or "but" or "and." Use the following strategy to deal with another person's anger:

A) Decide quickly that you will not get caught up in the other person's anger. Try to remember to take a deep breath and realize that the anger belongs completely to the other person, that no one else in the world can reach inside your brain and make you be angry. You choose your own behavior.

B) Acknowledge that you accept the fact that the angry person's feelings are real and/or valid, and that you hear and understand what the person is saying.

C) Admit that you feel defensive and upset that the anger is being directed at you.

D) Ask the angry person to clarify his or her position by giving you examples. Ask the person to explain what he or she means by certain words being used.

E) Diagnose the reasons for the anger and separate out the different causative factors. Asking the other person to speak more slowly so you can write down each of the points and concerns being expressed ("to make sure not to miss anything important") will often quiet the storm all by itself. This is an especially helpful step because most angry outbursts are accompanied by a barrage of complaints that seldom hold up to individual scrutiny once they are identified, listed, sorted out, and addressed.

F) Focus on renegotiating both the situation and the relationship by talking only about the issues involved.

G) Follow up the confrontation promptly. Don't allow time for things to "simmer." Within reason, do what you can to rebuild the bridge.

According to Jim Maselko of Designed Learning, Inc., a management training company for "Fortune 500" executives, virtually all anger "is triggered by a real or perceived threat, a real or perceived injustice, or by unmet expectations." One other form of anger, anger at oneself, is, says Maselko, "self-punishment for not meeting expectations set at some point in your life — often the result of parental messages we absorb in childhood: 'Be perfect.' 'Be strong.' 'Please everybody.' 'Hurry up.' 'Try hard.' Getting angry at oneself can block conflict resolution. If you're going to move forward in reaching some resolution, it's important to 'own' the anger, to acknowledge your inability to meet the demands of self-imposed expectations, and to forgive yourself."

When you're in a conflict situation, you're part of it. When you're part of it, you need to act. If you're going to act, act positively and responsibly. If you reach a point where you feel overwhelmed, Maselko advises workshop participants to simply "Throw your hands up in the air and call, 'Time out!'"

XVI

DR. BUSTED &
DR. MALPRACTICE:
SPECIALISTS IN
GENERAL OVERSIGHTS

Dealing With The SBE, PRO, FDA, IRS
(and Other Government Trappers)

As if it wasn't enough that you have chosen a profession that requires you to be ruled and regulated and policed and policed more frequently than most other professionals, you also must interact more often with governing and government body agents and employees, or "trappers."

Trappers are the people who slink around in the shadows of your practice, waiting to lunge out at you from the dark during your most vulnerable moment. Trappers work for government regulatory agencies or for state examiner boards or peer review organizations. Regardless of employer, there's very little discernable difference between individual trappers.

Trappers often have no patience and little mercy. The best way to deal with trappers is to not deal with them at all. You're a doctor, not a lawyer, arbitrator, auctioneer, lion tamer, or snake charmer. Let your lawyer do the communicating; that's what he or she is there for. The other secret to dealing with trappers is to keep your focus on the present, the "here and now." Take lots of deep breaths. Trappers will try to keep you focused on the past. If they win at this, you lose.

Focusing On The Present

Should you have any doubts about the value of staying mentally alert and focused on the "here and now" to avoid getting "zapped," perhaps you will appreciate an anecdote taken from *It Isn't This Time of Year at*

All: An Unpremeditated Autobiography (Doubleday, New York, 1954) by
Dr. Oliver St. John Gogarty. The controversial Irish poet/author/surgeon,
host to James Joyce, Samuel Beckett, and the Churchills among many
prominent friends, writes of a Patient examination in his home office,
with side comments about two of his literary companions, Sir Thomas
Moore and W.B. Yeats:

> At home I found a woman waiting, in a downstairs room, to
> be transilluminated; that is, examined for sinusitis by a lighted
> electric lamp placed in the patient's mouth in a dark room. (If
> there were to be a denture or upper plate, it must be first
> removed.) When it is being transilluminated, the face looks like
> 'a face carved out of a turnip,' as Yeats described the face of
> Moore. Don't get the impression that Yeats was vindictive. He
> would never have made that remark had not Moore first
> described him as looking like an umbrella forgotten at a picnic.
> This is an aside.
>
> While the eight-volt lamp was in the seated patient's mouth,
> I had the misfortune to touch a hand-basin full of water. Instantly
> I was flung down and spread-eagled upon the floor. I had
> grounded the electric wire and sent the town's uninterrupted
> current of more than two hundred volts into my chest. I was all
> but electrocuted. I remember thinking of the agony of
> electrocuted persons. At last the flex broke: I was saved. Oh, the
> relief! A voice from the chair inquired anxiously, 'Oh, Doctor,
> am I as bad as that?'

As Dr. Gogarty learned, you must be cognizant of the misfortunes of
not keeping total concentration on the here and now. Why all this
emphasis on staying focused on the present? Because answering
government, peer review, or state board charges is the one time in your
life when a good offense is not the best defense. In fact, any kind of
offense will almost always ignite a self-destructive fuse.

Remember, you're dealing with people who would like nothing better
than for you to lose control. This could prove their point that you are
prone to losing control and reacting poorly under stress. *You lose control
the minute you move your mind into the past or future without exercising
control of those past or future thoughts from a position of constant
present awareness.* What will help you most to stay in control in the here
and now? Are you breathing?

Steven Kern, the top physicians' advocacy attorney for the New York and New Jersey Medical Societies tells the following story of an actual case experience when asking doctors to consider how safe they may be from government abuses. According to Kern, stories such as this one are all too common:

A 72-year-old senile dement was admitted to the hospital suffering from dehydration. At the time of admission, the E.R. physician ordered an SMA which reported a Hemoglobin of 4.8 and a hematocrit of 14.5. The panic value system at the hospital failed, no nurse picked up on the abnormal result, and, indeed, the quality assurance people missed it.

The attending mentally transposed the two values when looking at the lab report and, therefore, did not realize the problem. The patient was discharged and then readmitted two weeks later for anemia. She was transfused and again discharged, without sequelae.

The PRO found this to be a 'gross and flagrant' violation and then gave the doctor an opportunity to try to talk them out of it. Unlike any other area of law, in this arena, you are first found guilty and then given an opportunity to *attempt* to defend yourself. 'Innocent until proven guilty' does not apply to the PRO's.

In fact, the right to a full adversarial hearing does not exist until *after* the imposition of sanctions against the physician.

In other words, first you are found guilty, then you are punished, and while you are serving your sentence you *may* have a hearing to determine whether, in fact, you are guilty.

Equally sacred constitutional protection, including the right to know and confront your accusers, are uniformly denied. Not only can you not cross-examine the individuals who determined that your conduct constituted a gross and flagrant violation, the PRO's will not even provide you with the identity of these individuals.

Likewise, the PRO's do not wish the public to have knowledge of their activities. They ask that you, your experts, and your attorney sign a confidentiality oath before the process begins wherein you promise not to disclose anything that occurred during the hearing.... As far as I am concerned, the PRO's are attempting to use the issue of patient confidentiality as a vehicle to preclude the medical community from knowing what goes on behind closed doors.

This story is not intended to raise levels of paranoia. Rather, it is included more as a wake up call to reinforce the idea that government overregulation is a fact of life for doctors, and the only effective way to deal with this reality is realistically. Trappers are trappers. You cannot afford to waste time and energy trying to undo what they do. Your best protection is an ounce of prevention — having a qualified attorney with doctor advocacy experience standing ready in the wings to represent your interests.

Advisor Shopping

Similarly, a qualified accountant (you may have to shop long and hard for one who will serve as a guide instead of in the traditional role of historian) should be able to help you weave your way through the mind-boggling masses of tax laws and regulations. A reputable, doctor-experienced financial advisor (this could be the same person as your accountant) should be able to help you plan your cash flow to contend with the sea of government bureaucracy that carries the seemingly rudderless ships of Medicare and Medicaid, among other interests, through sporadic and erratic payment periods.

Finally, but perhaps most importantly, you need to find a doctor-experienced practice development/management/marketing consultant who knows when to be conservative on issues that border legal or government involvement (for example, that generic practice names in some states must include individual doctor/director names in all advertising). This individual must be accepted by your front desk people, and know how to train/retrain them in in-person and telephone Patient relations and in how to avoid malpractice-baited comments. This individual must also understand and practice effective human resource management.

Your consultant should deal with you in a direct manner, and be more concerned with growing your practice than with winning local advertising and design awards. He or she should take the initiative to act on your behalf when opportunities for image-building arise. The consultant is both a team player who can work harmoniously with your other advisors, associates, and staff people (and your spouse!) and a leader who will guide you through your business decision-making. She or he must be ethical to a fault.

When you have assembled the best team of advisors you can find and afford, let them do their jobs. Demand performance. Demand results. Make yourself available to them when they need you, but let them do what they do best (what they are paid to do) without your interference. Be realistic about the fact that doing their jobs right means taking longer than you would probably prefer or imagine. If you don't think you can trust a member of this team, find a replacement.

Ways I will start now to build or rebuild preventive layers of protection against the ever present dangers of malpractice suits and interventions from government and other regulatory organizations:

_____

_____

_____

_____

_____

_____

_____

_____

_____

_____

_____

_____

In case you didn't fill in any of the lines, you may want to give some thought to the fact that even if you survive the Trappers, you are not likely to avoid a malpractice suit. And the result, as far as you're concerned, is the same. Litigation can literally tear apart your insides.

Malpractice Stress

"It is the challenge to the personal integrity of the professional that is at the center of the malpractice stress syndrome," notes Rev. Edward G. Reading, head of the Litigation Stress Support Group, a New Jersey Medical Society program, in a March, 1987 *Maryland Medical Journal* article entitled "Malpractice Stress Syndrome: A New Diagnosis?" "Physicians take suits as personal attacks, and the resulting stress can be crippling," says Reading in an article entitled "The Proven Ways To Deal With Malpractice Stress," in the July, 1990 edition of *Medical Economics*.

Rev. Reading also reports, "Because doctors are generally unable to separate who they are from what they do, they feel tremendous stress when they're accused of making a serious professional mistake." He cites feelings of shame, anger, isolation, and negative self-image as precursors to a long list of physical and psychological symptoms that evolve in malpractice stress cases. His eleven "portions" of "food for thought" are:

1. **Don't overwork.** Many doctors try to avoid their problems by increasing their already heavy workload — which increases stress.

2. **Don't self-prescribe or self-medicate.** This includes alcohol, pharmaceuticals, and illegal drugs. If you really need help, see a psychiatrist or psychologist, and don't think it means you're a head case; it's just good healthcare.

3. **Don't isolate yourself or your family.** Stay active with professional and social support systems. It's at this time that you'll find out who your real friends are.

4. **Maintain a low-stress comfort level at home.** Talk things out with your spouse. As often as possible, discuss your feelings about being sued.

5. **Don't discuss the case itself with anyone but your spouse, your attorney, or the insurance company rep.** If the plaintiff's lawyer learns that you discussed specifics of the case with your friends and colleagues, he could depose them and use the testimony against you.

6. **Learn conflict-resolution skills.** Know when to fight, when to negotiate, and when to go with the flow.

7. **Learn to identify your mood cycles and to recognize situations that anger you.**

8. **Clarify your values and priorities in both your personal and professional life.**

9. **Learn and practice relaxation skills such as yoga and meditation.**

10. **It helps to have a spiritual anchor.**

11. **Confront your fear of the litigation process.**

Preparing For Court

Now that the nasty subject of malpractice litigation is out on the table, an enormously helpful article to review is "Judges Tell How to Win — or Lose — A Malpractice Trial," which appeared in the July, 1993 *Medical Economics For Surgeons* and was written by Senior Editor Brad Burg. When the fearful, god-awful moment arrives, be aware that Burg's interviews with a cross-section of malpractice-experienced judges point up "It's not just your testimony that sways a jury. What can be equally important are factors doctors may never think of." Here are some of those critically important and often overlooked considerations.

"Not all good malpractice attorneys are good malpractice *trial* attorneys," says Burg, who supports this point with testimony from San Francisco jurist Alan W. Haverty. Haverty advises finding "a specialist in the type case against you," and notes, "I know of lawyers who are experts in 'failure to diagnose breast cancer.'" Former trial court judge H. Warren Knight advises doctors to not meekly accept their insurance company's choice of a lawyer if it's someone the doctor doesn't feel confident in, even though the choice may not technically be theirs.

As for preparation, Burg cites Judge Johanna Fitzpatrick, who is now on Virginia's Appellate Court after ten years as a trial judge: "I sometimes see doctors who count too much on their attorneys to know all the details of the case. You," she tells doctors, "are the main expert for your side. Be thoroughly familiar with all the facts and records, or you may be unpleasantly surprised on the stand." Houston Judge Sharolyn P. Wood adds that doctors must review every word of their depositions to avoid being misled by disarming questions from opposing lawyers who seek to discredit the doctor by making him or her appear to be lying.

Judge Richard S. Dodge of Dayton, Ohio, recommends practicing cross-examination with one of your lawyer's partners, preferably someone who's tough, and whom you haven't met. Also, spend time in the courtroom beforehand as an observer. Burg's interview with New York Judge Ira Gammerman produced the following assessment: "Even a brilliant doctor needs to know how to behave in court. I once had a very prominent young physician lose a close one, but it didn't surprise me. He was cocky, hostile to the plaintiff's attorneys, even rude to me. I think he learned from it though. Two years later, I heard another case against him, and I'd have sworn his evil twin had been at the other trial. This time he couldn't have been more personable and gracious. It was a close case again; this time he won."

Other jurist advice extracted by Burg:

- *Anticipate a hard time.* Prepare to be challenged and have your reputation questioned. Don't take it personally and stay calm.

- *Don't be arrogant.* Judges generally agree that this is the doctor's biggest trap in testifying. Remember, jurors will forgive an arrogant attorney because they know it's part of the job. They won't forgive your arrogance; it's inappropriate (the same goes for sarcasm).

- *Know you can get help.* If you do feel squeezed, don't panic. You may get help from the bench. Browbeating and physical crowding are part of the game. Don't hesitate to ask the judge for help (including a rest room break if you don't feel well) if your lawyer doesn't ask.

- *Keep your answers narrow.* Houston's Judge Wood says, "If you mention the wrong topic, the plaintiff's attorney will pick up that ball and run with it. For example, Texas courts, like many other state courts, don't permit discussions of your finances and insurance. But suppose a lawyer suggests you do unnecessary procedures, and in replying you say, 'I don't need to make money that way; I do very well.' Now you've raised the issue, and your entire financial picture is fair game."

- *Simply looking right is also important.* Dress conservatively and without flashy jewelry. Leave the golf shirt, expensive watch, snazzy tie, and even your expensive car at home.

- *The trial doesn't start and stop at the courtroom door.* You're on trial in the hallways and on the front steps, too. You'll be noticed in the parking lot or at the coffee shop, when you least expect it. A plaintiff's attorney, plaintiff's attorney's assistant, or a juror's glimpses of you and your "off the stand" behavior can make unfair but lasting impressions that will sometimes have more to do with your fate than what takes place in the courtroom.

In a nutshell, when on the stand: Be clear. Address the jury. Keep it simple. Be professional. Be yourself. Be present even when you're not required to be. Invite your spouse to show up — don't be afraid to show your family (jurors can't relate to being doctors, but they can relate to your human side).

Justice Knight told Burg, "From the first day in court, keep in mind that it's the plaintiff who must prove the case. I'll watch a doctor start to sweat as everything his experts have said is contradicted 100% by the other side, and he wonders who the jury will believe. But he would suffer less if he remembered that the plaintiff has the burden of proof; so if the jury's confused about who's right, they have to vote in his favor. That's one reason many verdicts go for doctors. To find for the doctor, the jury doesn't have to be sure there was no malpractice. They only have to be not sure there was any."

Judge Wood concluded, "Even with everybody's best intentions, a trial doesn't determine the ultimate truths of a case. So a verdict against you simply means that most of the evidence, as presented in this one room, to this jury, was in the plaintiff's favor. Don't take it as indicating you're a bad doctor. Only you know in your heart how well you did your job."

XVII

HOW TO STOP WISHING YOU COULD DO MORE FOR PATIENTS

Patients want doctors who do what they say they're going to do. This means keeping your word as well as keeping your appointments. This also means you would do well to assess the extent to which the habits you practice and patterns you follow are fostering Patient acceptance. Can you rearrange your life enough to move business/investment meetings and phone calls out of the mainstream traffic of Patient office hours? Patients will accept, respect, and trust you more when you don't interrupt or delay your time with them for the sake of your personal or business interests.

Similarly, Patients don't want to hear or overhear office chatter about your big house, your new car, your stocks and bonds, where you send your children to school, or how luxurious your vacation was or will be. Make certain your staff people know this. For the same reason that retail stores have quietly moved to quieter cash registers (besides quieter technology), and muffled register sounds with piped-in music — to avoid reminding shoppers that they're spending money — you don't need to be reminding Patients of what they already believe is too high a price to pay for your services. You also *definitely* don't need to be reminding them of the impression that they might in any way be paying for your new Mercedes or ski house, your recent trip to Hawaii, or for your daughter to go to Princeton.

Study reports and articles are filled with cases that clearly show Patients want reassurance even more than solutions. A comprehensive Patient study done by one hospital, and supported by informal reports from at least three others, reveals that an estimated 80% of all hospital visits, including those to the E.R., are made in search of reassurance! "You're going to be just fine; the tetanus shot will prevent blood poisoning and the antiseptic and bandage will help keep the wound clean; take a couple of aspirin if it hurts tonight and call me in the morning so we can check on how you're doing, okay?"

Reassurance may not seem so important to you, but — to a patient — reassurance of good health, of quick recovery, of total recovery, sometimes even reassurance of just partial recovery can be more desirable than an actual solution. So keep in mind that communicating *some* form of reassurance is almost always a valuable thing to do, and it is almost always possible, even when solutions may not be. Most medical schools now readily acknowledge the need for more Patient communications training aimed at teaching doctors how to talk with Patients; how much to listen, how much to say, and how to feel more confident about what to say regardless of the circumstances.

"In such a litigious society as we have, I've become very hesitant to speak freely with patients. This is especially true with respect to what I would perceive their odds to be for success with certain procedures, and this is something practically everyone seems to ask about at some point for either themselves or others," admits a leading anesthesiologist, whose comments are echoed by many doctors.

How can you improve your efforts to provide more of the reassurance that Patients seek? Begin by asking more personal, more pointed questions to get answers that will help you learn more about each Patient's work and home environment, lifestyle, stress factors, and support relationships. Then be sure to listen attentively! When you find yourself getting bored or impatient with the answers offered, *question your questions.* Ask about things that interest you, things that you genuinely want to learn more about. Ask for information that will help you size up, or discover more of the environment that surrounds this body you're examining or treating. Why? Because you can never offer someone any meaningful degree of reassurance without first knowing some of the significant factors that make that person tick.

When you're concerned that the answers your questions might generate could be too long and drawn out for the time available, ask more pointed, closed-end questions that set the stage for prompting concise and direct responses. Instead of asking the general question "What do you like to do in your free time?" try rephrasing the question to ask "What three things do you most enjoy doing on weekends?" The answers to this question will indicate a Patient's personal interests, lifestyle, and activity level. You'll certainly want to consider differences in treatment, for example, for a construction worker who enjoys running 10-15 miles on weekends as opposed to a computer operator who prefers 10-15 hours of reading books on weekends.

Try questions that will reveal "a different side" of the Patient. Such insight may provide some common ground for relating to each other, or give you a better feel for ways to present medical examples, analogies, and treatment direction information. One example of such a question is: "Do you have a pet at home? What's the funniest thing it does?" Pets are proven to be good therapy, especially for most kinds of rehabilitation. Just thinking and talking about them is therapeutic in that it relieves stress. Getting a Patient to focus on something humorous about the pet will relieve stress even further.

"The responses I get to this question," says a prominent osteopath, "never cease to amaze and entertain me. I learn so much more about a patient's character makeup. The answers give me lots of clues about which treatment options might work best...how much more patience, for example, a person has who regularly breeds puppies than someone who just tends to a stray cat, or who has no pets. Rehab potential is reflected here."

The kind of question everyone likes to answer can be very telling as to a Patient's personal goals, strength of support relationships, sense of independence, and energy level, all of which can affect treatment adherence as well as results. "If you could take an all-expenses-paid vacation anywhere in the world, where would you go? When would you go? Why? Who would you take? How would you spend your time?" Although the answers this short series of questions may prompt are likely to be a bit more lengthy than the previous examples, getting the Patient to fantasize a bit helps reduce some of the immediate stress of having to see you. In addition, the answers can actually tell you everything you really need to know about your Patient's likes, dislikes, lifestyle, value and support system, activity interests and levels, etc.

Ask. Listen. Observe. Process the information. Once again, be a detective. Remember that your personal goal when preparing for each Patient visit should be to help the Patient reduce her or his stress and resistance levels as quickly as possible to facilitate your examination or treatment. Sometimes this occurs through the use of humor, other times by prompting pleasant memories. It can almost always be attained with a combination of deep breathing and fantasizing, e.g., "So how about taking a deep breath, and then tell me what you're going to do if you win the lottery tomorrow."

The caring doctor frequently stands torn between subjective feelings and objective reality. Part of the problem is that there are no rules for how to communicate with Patients and Patient families. Depending on circumstances, the mind often speaks what the heart and soul would prefer not to say. Sharing feelings, emotions, and beliefs with Patients may simply be inviting unnecessary risk. By the same token, absorbing too many Patient fears and upsets can also put your performance at risk.

Where to Draw the Proverbial Line_____?

Martha Weinman Lear, in her *New York Times Magazine* article (January 24, 1993), "Should Doctors Tell The Truth?," says, "Today, unvarnished truth seems to have yielded to what one doctor calls 'a *slightly* varnished truth,' by which he means not a lie but a good spin on bad news. As in: A patient comes to Dr. Ronald Weintraub (chief of cardiothoracic surgery) at Beth Israel (Hospital in Boston) as a candidate for open heart surgery. He is too high-risk and is turned down."

"Dr. Weintraub says: 'The absolute truth would have been to say (that) you are so sick and your heart is so bad that if I operate on you, I'll kill you. Instead, I said: I've looked at the alternatives. Surgery would carry high risk and I think that, in your situation, continued medical therapy is the way to go. It's euphemism, sure. He was sent to me because medicines weren't working well anymore. But you don't need to hit people over the head.'"

Lear's article supports Weintraub's reasoning with comments from Dr. James F. Holland, an oncologist and chairman of the Department of Neoplastic Diseases at Mount Sinai Medical Center in New York, who agrees: "Say a patient asks, 'Do I have a chance?' It serves no useful purpose to say, 'Yes, about one in a hundred' though that may be statistically so. But it *is* useful to say, 'Yes, but you must work for it, because the treatment won't be easy.' Then they concentrate on the positive elements of treatment. People need the possibility of hope."

"It might be called the 'Bad News, But' school of truth-telling: 'The treatment hasn't worked, *but* we never know what's just around the corner.'"

There seems, incidentally, to be no corner on the market of bad taste and bad judgement communications, long thought to be limited to those doctors who deal only with adult-level traumas. One spinal surgeon's last words outside the O.R. to the anxiety-ridden parents of a severely injured eight-year-old girl who had been hit by a car were: "Look, I do this all the time. If she doesn't make it, I'll kill myself, alright?"

Even if this statement had been made in jest (which it was not), even if the parents' hysteria had been disrupting the entire nurses' station (which it was not), even if the doctor had been up all night, had a fight with his wife, had stubbed his toe on the curb, and gotten a flat tire on his way to the hospital (which he hadn't), there simply are no circumstances to justify a comment like that. Imagine how *you* would feel. So much, you see, of being a doctor has to do with imagining how you would feel as a Patient.

Flash Yourself!

To better imagine how you would feel as your own Patient, try this: Flash yourself! Not open-raincoat-in-front-of-a-mirror style, but mentally. If for just one fraction of an instant before opening your mouth to a troubled Patient or Patient friend or family member, you flash through your mind a quick picture of what it might be like to be standing in their shoes, looking to you for answers, you will probably say something much more comforting, reassuring, and professional than you would have without the "flash." By forcing yourself to do this, you will *also* be forcing yourself to pause before responding, and that, all by itself, is a comforting behavior in the Patient's eyes because it communicates that you are giving serious, thoughtful attention to her or his needs.

There's no doubt about it, doctor, that in spite of what the world would have had you believe in the past, and what you may believe the world still believes, you are not God! As one member of what has traditionally been considered an exclusive healthcare fraternity, you can only undo the negative characteristics commonly ascribed to doctors nowadays by undoing the attachment of these attributes to you individually. In other words, to have any impact on the public's rapidly deteriorating image of your profession (which, in turn, is damaging to you as a member of it), you must consciously strive to serve as an example of the positive characteristics.

As Associate Dean of Student Affairs for Columbia University's College of Physicians and Surgeons, Dr. Linda Lewis is quoted in a November 28, 1993 *New York Times* article by Elisabeth Rosenthal, titled "How Doctors Learn To Think They're DOCTORS." Dr. Lewis is reported as saying "...patients have become more sophisticated, the aloof attitude that may have served doctors well in the past is now dysfunctional. 'Doctors have been patronizing and paternalistic, I think, because they were mostly men who looked at their patients as their children. Patients have become very bright and physicians being so conservative have not caught up to that.'"

Dr. Lewis' reminder to new doctor graduates that their white coats were "cloaks of compassion...symbols to remind them of the importance of humility in their careers" is juxtaposed with author Rosenthal's comment, "But to the public, those white coats have also at times come to symbolize the arrogance and greed of an exclusive fraternity."

You may find yourself still being thought of as an omnipotent being by some people, but be careful not to believe or reinforce that image. Times have changed. To succeed, and to continue to succeed, you can no longer act out the fantasy of unrealistic roles that were associated with your profession in the past. You must be willing to assume some degree of humility and accept the fact that you are no longer considered to be all things by all people.

The odds are that, far from being omnipotent, your "self" is not even healthy or physically fit. Setting aside any possible addictive/self-destructive behaviors, you still may be among the frailest of human beings, given your constant exposure to mental and emotional stress, physical infections and ill health, and the poor diet and low fitness levels doctors typically subject themselves to in the race to serve and/or profit by their Patients.

It's your perseverance, ambition, industriousness, entrepreneurship, drive, resilience, dedication to healing (and in varying degrees, wellness), commitment to education, skilled hands and eyes, and strong sense of responsibility that carry you through the day-to-day challenges in your personal and professional lives.

Despite all these positive attributes, you suffer for the Patients you think you've failed, and for the Patients for whom your every ounce of courage, skill, and empathy could make no difference. Yet from all this conflict between doubt and confidence, ignorance and wisdom, naivete and experience, in this arena of riches and poverty of life, emerges the awareness that a set of realistic expectations must go hand in hand with a solid professional competency.

What is Possible?

It is said Einstein only used 10% of his brain, and that if humans could utilize 100% of the brain's power, it would allow for the possibility of separating molecules to be able to walk through a wall. What is possible?

What percentage of the time do you think your ability to turn in a top-notch, A-1 Patient diagnostic or treatment performance is truly limited by what you know and don't know, by what you do and don't do? What percentage could be reversed by you by teaching Patients how to behave as responsible "investor/partners," working in concert with you, your Staff, and others to expedite delivery of their own healthcare needs or preservation of their own wellness programs?

Isn't it true that the elusive "more" that you could do for Patients, which is clearly the option that makes the most sense, is to help your Patients take greater responsibility for working with you to get better and stay better?

If your answer is "Yes, but...," you are essentially saying that:

A) Since Patients can only take more responsibility by being more assertive than you probably like, you are afraid to let go of your presumed controls;

B) Your ego is bigger and more important than your Patient's desire for expedited healthcare delivery;

C) You don't trust your Patients to do their share and be able to act responsibly;

D) You don't believe your Patients have the awareness or sophistication levels you believe are necessary to act responsibly;

E) You think people simply don't care to be involved in the process. People just want you to fix them up, make them better, or get them out functioning and "back to normal" without having to participate, without having to think, without having to work, and without wanting to know all the details;

F) Other_____

_____

_____.

Circle or underline the parts of A, B, C, D, E, and F that apply to your way of thinking right now. Follow up with a statement that relates your choices above to the thinking/feeling behaviors you believe might be in your own best interest to begin cultivating right now. A single sentence is fine, but try to phrase it as a goal and in the present tense (e.g., "Right now I am working harder to teach my Patients how to accept greater responsibility for adhering to my prescriptions and heeding my advice.")

_____

_____

_____

Could it be that your convictions are unjustly tainted by your own presumptions and prejudices? To paraphrase a major-impact old song title (*Give Peace A Chance*), perhaps you need to:

Give P's (for "Patients") A Chance

Patient empowerment-themed books and articles are fraught with references to "Patient Partnerships." It's already beyond counting how many hospitals are actively engaged in marketing "Partners In Health" types of themes, though very few seem to actually produce much more than promotional clamor.

This translates to: You're in the middle of a lot of noise about Patient Partnerships. The tendency is to cover your ears until things quiet down. The reality is, things won't quiet down. You must begin to shift gears *now*, take a leadership posture, learn more about empowerment (check current management text books, articles, and seminars), and begin to practice empowerment approaches *now*, with both Staff and Patients.

Empowering others means helping them to take greater responsibility (a greater sense of *ownership*) for those parts of their lives or careers that are rightfully theirs to begin with. We empower ourselves and others, says Peter Block in his book *The Empowered Manager* (Jossey-Bass, 1987), "by compulsively asking the question 'if this is what we have to get done, what do you want from me and others to make it happen?'" Block lists four ways to help replace sacrifice with the commitment that's called for by empowerment:

1) At the simplest level, stay focused on what we and those around us want.

2) Act in ways that give others ownership. We create ownership/commitment when we give others freedom to choose their own path to achieving results, and when we structure work so that people are doing a whole job instead of a piece of a job.

3) Discourage and confront passive, nonassertive behavior. Passive people remain silent as a strategy for getting what they want by making others feel either guilty or sorry for them.

4) Create a vision of greatness for ourselves and ask our subordinates to do the same.

At a Patient level, this means keeping tuned in to what the *Patient* wants (vs. what you want for the Patient). It means *involving* the Patient in both diagnostic and treatment decision-making. For example, consider encouraging the *Patient* to choose between comparable drugs with different side effects (regardless of which detail rep you prefer or which manufacturer provides more sporting event tickets). Consider encouraging the *Patient* to decide on the pros and cons of an x-ray, MRI, or CT scan after explaining your recommendation and reasons.

It means that you need to encourage each Patient to think and communicate more assertively with you, to speak up and ask questions, to even research something for themselves. It means helping each Patient to visualize her or himself as having reached a goal that he or she has set, to improve, feel better, return to normalcy, excel in performance, etc., and to continue helping each person to see and strive for that goal.

XVIII

A VIEW FROM THE HOSPITAL COFFEE SHOP

The Doctor/Hospital Cold War

"I frequently do several surgeries a day, but I could probably do twice as many if the hospital administrative line wasn't so long and padded...doctors simply can't get through it to get quick decisions."
— A doctor

"I planned a complex surgical procedure that necessitated various companies bringing specialized equipment, and grafting tissue, into the hospital. Everything was set in advance. The patient arrived on time and was fully prepped and premedicated. As I was about to start, I saw that the consent form, which is legal for a maximum of one month, was executed three months earlier. The on-call nurse explained that an administrator told her he didn't think it would be necessary to get a new form. We couldn't exactly wake the patient to have a new form signed and then put him back to sleep...and I wasn't about to take the liability risk on my own shoulders. Everything had to be undone. What a huge waste of time and effort, not to mention the resultant stress and upsets experienced by the poor victimized patient and his anxious family. Unfortunately, situations like this occur all too often."
— A doctor

"I've heard endless horror stories of patient suffering brought on by inept hospital administrators, and how it's always the hospitals that are at fault, but — deep down inside — I know most of that is bull. It's almost always the doctor's fault when equipment is not checked out and functioning properly, or when something is not communicated clearly.

"We're human; that makes us not perfect; the problem is doctors are overloaded with responsibility to begin with...and we don't like the guilt feelings or ego upsets that go along with screwing up.... In the end, though, it's worse to blame someone else than it is to actually screw up, and own it."

— A doctor

Operating flaws are causing many MDs to give up on hospitals entirely; surgeons taking all or part of their outpatient cases away from hospitals cite poor operations as the 'trigger' for defection.

— The Advisory Board Company consulting firm in "SURGERY: Executive Introduction To Leading Hospital Strategies," a heavily-documented summary of a two-part, three-volume set of studies and plans for re-engineering hospital O.R.'s.

"The day is not so far away when hospitals, because they have not responded quickly, enthusiastically, and businesslike enough to the rapid economical, technological, and societal shifts occurring, will only be the dwelling place of extremely sick people. We are going to see much more emphasis on wellness environments and preventive medicine. Hospitals simply don't make it when it comes to meeting the growing demands for this wellness/preventive level of health care."

— A doctor

November 27, 1993...Worcester, Massachusetts — A state medical board has fined a surgeon and an anesthesiologist $10,000 each and ordered them to undergo joint psychotherapy, in addition to five years of probation monitoring, for brawling in an operating room while their patient slept under general anesthesia.

The anesthesiologist reportedly swore at the surgeon, who threw a cotton-tipped prep stick in rebuttal. The two then raised their fists and scuffled briefly, at one point wrestling on the floor while a nurse monitored the anesthetized patient. The two later completed the half hour surgery successfully...

— Associated Press

"You just tell us, Doctor, what you would like done here at the hospital and we'll see to it that it happens. It's our job to make you happy. We want to help you because we realize that it's the only way we can be successful. If you're not satisfied, you won't bring your patients here, and if you don't bring your patients here, well, you know the rest, Doctor. So tell us, Doctor, what you would like done here and..."
— A hospital administrator

"Of course we are *trying*, Doctor, to actually implement some of those ideas you had when we met last year. In fact, since that time, we actually went out and hired a consultant to help us figure out the best way to get started. The consultant is already halfway through a feasibility study to determine how you and the other doctors can help the hospital to streamline some of the coding policies we use so you don't have to spend so much time working on patient charts! And, oh yes, we're still assessing some of the other points you raised, so it won't be much longer now before you start to see some real results..."
— A hospital administrator

"The doctors here are a pain in the ass. All they ever want is more, more, more. They're never satisfied."
— A hospital administrator

"Hospitals continue to be insensitive places that employ insensitive people to deal with sensitive needs and situations. How much more cockamamie can anything be?"
— A doctor

Take the issues raised by these eight quotes and two print excerpts and put them together. What have you got? Confusion. Yet there is a common denominator. Throughout all these diverse items and issues, there surfaces the basic principle of all practice and professional development, the single unifying thread that weaves through every aspect of doctor/doctor relations, doctor/hospital relations, doctor/Patient relations, doctor/Staff relations, doctor/family relations and doctor/community relations: Communication.

Rising or falling on the strength or weakness of these areas of communication match-ups are the strengths and weaknesses of every doctor's relations with his or her hospital(s). Expert testimony and textbook suggestions not withstanding, it is quite difficult to communicate too much. "Not so," you say, because you know someone who does talk too much, and you also know some doctors who overindulge in both Patient conversations and technical explanations.

Over-communicating in casual conversation or in offering some technical explanation is not uncommon, granted, but over-communicating in giving someone directions is rare. This is especially true in diagnostic and treatment settings, such as in describing exactly what instruments are needed in the O.R., what exact angle to use for an x-ray, how many units of what should be prepared for an injection, how many minutes/hours/ times per day someone needs to follow a prescription or prescribed treatment, or what specific notations need to appear on a Patient's chart. These types of details are rarely given too much attention.

If anything is done "too much," by the way, it's probably too much assuming that others (even those you may have worked with for years) are as sharp and tuned in as you are, which *may* be too big of an assumption. That others are easily able to understand your mumbling is *probably* too big of an assumption. That others fully understand your scribbling and your abbreviations is *almost certainly* too much to assume, according to published reports.

For practically any type of doctor, a typical case can easily involve as many as 100 or more little decisions involving scheduling and diagnostic testing alone. A single miscommunication or a single unspoken detail is all it takes to cost major chunks of time, money, aggravation, and quality of care. How are miscommunications best avoided? With concentrated effort to listen "between the lines," and, when in doubt, talk too much! Overkill with detail, and request lots of feedback, confirmation, and paraphrasing. How else can you be reasonably sure that you're clearly understood?

And when was the last time you actually sat down with the appropriate hospital administrator(s) to discuss your ideas or concerns for making some kind of policy or procedural improvement? Do you know for a fact, for instance, that the hospital is using the most effective methods or products at the best dollar value? Can you suggest ways to cut costs without cutting quality? Do you make value-conscious suggestions like this? Have you made them in the past? Are you putting off or holding back from having this kind of meeting because you think no one will pay attention, or because you haven't the time, or because you only know what's wrong but not how to fix it, or because you figure it's not your job? Are you making excuses for not acting like a leader or a team player? Can you do something more positive about your procrastination (or, your imagination, as the case may be) this week? What? Spell it out:

_____

_____

_____

_____

_____

_____

_____

_____

_____

Who can you call right now, today, to set up an appointment for discussing areas of improvement with the hospital(s), surgical center(s), urgent care center(s), or other institution(s) or institutional program(s) you are presently involved with, or plan to be involved with in the near future? Jot down who to call and what to talk about:

_____

_____

_____

_____

_____

_____

_____

_____

_____

Toward these same ends, one thing you might suggest to your hospital administrator(s) is that the hospital initiate a Doctors' Focus Group Roundtable; a discussion group to meet once a month (even quarterly is a good start) with an agenda driven by the desire for input and ideas about particular areas of improvement that the doctors perceive to be in need of attention. You might also suggest a similar group meeting approach for Patients to address current issues involving Patient care. Most progressive nursing homes meet regularly with resident family member groups for this purpose. Most doctors could stand to benefit by doing this for themselves as well.

One doctor monitors and adjusts her practice by having her practice manager meet regularly to solicit one hour's worth of input and ideas from five people: two past Patients and three current Patients (all are encouraged to bring along a friend or spouse for a five to ten-minute "Speak Out" portion of the meeting where guests are urged to contribute any thoughts they had while they quietly observed the first 50 minutes). The group's composition changes with each meeting. Patient Advisory Council Members, as they're called, are each given a small table plant arrangement and a personalized certificate of appreciation, signed by the doctor, as an expression of thanks for their time and opinions.

Quarterly focus group roundtable meetings of five Patients each = 20 plants and certificates a year = 20 objective, informed opinions from people who (just by virtue of having participated in the discussions) will often become your most exuberant supporters and referrers = 20 new opportunities a year to improve your practice in the eyes of those who matter most: your Patients!

Advisory Council discussions focus on the ways each participant thinks the doctor could improve her Patient relations skills, office administrative skills, scheduling, follow-up arrangements, Patient education approaches (and materials), written and telephone communications, and advertising messages. "It works like crazy," the doctor says, "even after ten years of practice; I never stop learning better ways to do things, and the meetings alone have a way of producing new Patients."

Of course this kind of program is rendered completely meaningless without a genuinely open-minded, responsive attitude on the doctor's part. *If the roundtable discussions produce ideas, the doctor must produce action on the ideas.* Action steps serve to set up yet another effective method of "Quiet Medical Marketing" (Chapter V).

Following up on the implementation of any ideas raised by these groups with personal thank you notes signed by the doctor (or "Honorable Mentions" in a practice newsletter, or both) helps secure increased Patient loyalties and additional referrals.

How to Function at Hospital Functions

Knowing how to function at hospital functions opens yet another "Quiet Medical Marketing" door to building referrals. If you don't know any 13-year-olds going on their first date, and you'd like to see a real live "study in awkwardness," watch some doctors try to function at a hospital function such as a fund-raising event. Better yet, watch their husbands and wives.

Whatever shreds of self-confidence you may possess, seem to dissolve when you suddenly find yourself surrounded by other doctors and spouses you don't know, and by hospital brass you do know, but would prefer not to, in the guise of a social setting that is actually just the wrapping for a business activity. And it's likely your wife or husband is light years less comfortable than you are.

So, what's the magic answer to feeling more comfortable? Are you breathing? *The key to making the most of hospital function functioning is, unfortunately, to not let your guard down.* Don't let the cocktails, munchies, music, laughter, and stress-free appearances disarm you. Business is business is business, even when it's disguised as a black tie ball with a dance band, entertainment, and party decorations. If you thought you could trip over a chair next to the dance floor and not have 20 people whisper about how much you must have had to drink, or that your wife could sashay across the room scantily dressed in a skintight sequined nothing (with nothing underneath) and have nothing derogatory said about *both* of you, you are sadly mistaken and lacking when it comes to good business sense. "Undoctor-like" and "undoctor-spouse-like" conduct will hardly have enhanced your ability to draw referrals from other doctors in attendance, and could actually end up costing you referrals from those who are not even present, who just *hear* about your stumble with drink in hand or your inappropriately dressed wife from those who are present.

Regardless of external appearances, treat every hospital-based activity as business. Don't choose to be drawn into letting your guard down by others who may be less savvy to the protocol, even when the "others" are the very same hospital people who are responsible for establishing and maintaining the behavioral guidelines to begin with. This doesn't mean you need to stand in a corner with your arms folded, holding a glass of milk and wearing a frown on your face, or that your wife needs to wear a body bag with a scarf wrapped around her head. It means simply that you must use good judgement about how you look and what you say. Just as Patients and Staff observe your every move in the office, hospital types (and other doctors) observe your every move at hospital-sponsored events and settings.

When you or your husband or wife don't fit the image others think you should have, you run the risk of losing their respect (as artificial as it may seem to you) and, thus, their referrals. When both of you do fit expectations, you increase the odds of generating continued or increased referrals. This is not just for points in a "game," it's for carrying the responsibilities you elected to carry by becoming a doctor, and by continuing to choose to carry them in this society.

Hospital social functions further dictate that you keep your conversations light and friendly. Your grandparents probably told you to steer clear of discussing politics and religion unless you're looking for a fight, but it's unlikely anyone in medical, dental or chiropractic school ever told you to avoid certain subjects and behaviors at hospital or other community-sponsored benefits and social gatherings. Do *not* talk shop! Do *not* talk business! Do *not* tell off-color jokes or stories! *Do not drink too much!* (If you make your first two drinks ginger ale, mineral water, or club soda, you won't be chugging wine, beer, or cocktails to quench your thirst.)

You needn't fumble around searching for conversational subject matter. Talk about books, movies, vacations, travel, music, pets, children (if you must), sports (if you must), but *not* Patients, *not* Staff, *not* other doctors, *not* new healthcare technologies/treatments/methods, *not* HMO's/PPO's/IPA's or seminars/journal articles/academy newsletters, *not* hospital or community politics/ policies/procedures/appointments. When you find your mouth starting to drift, rest it for a minute with a big deep breath, then return the conversation to something simple.

When others seek to draw you into business or shop talk discussions, pleasantly sidetrack the issue(s) into a suggested office, breakfast, lunch, or dinner meeting, and then move the conversation back to the books/movies line of topics. If you feel you're being sucked into the wrong conversation by others' insistence at staying with business, healthcare, or political subjects, simply excuse yourself. Community and hospital social events are neither the time nor the place for such discussions.

As for hospital functions that are not so camouflaged in social wraps and graces, such as departmental and committee meetings, be careful to walk the thin diplomatic line between over-committing yourself and not doing your share or asserting your ideas. When you volunteer to participate, you need to participate. If you think you're not going to have the time or energy to participate, don't volunteer in the first place. On the other hand, don't ignore or avoid involvement altogether. It's like politics; you can't complain about who gets elected if you didn't vote. There's not much you can say in criticism of hospital activities that you refused to discuss or failed to participate in when they were in the planning stages.

Not incidentally, this same thinking extends itself to the need for you to collect phone messages at least twice daily (hourly, and sometimes even more frequently in critical care situations), and pick up or arrange to have your hospital mail picked up at least once a week. It may be true that 98% of what gets jammed into your mailbox is a colossal waste of paper (perhaps something else to speak with administrators about), but the one time it will be very important for you to know something, the information will almost certainly be sitting quietly in your box during one of those intervals where you ignored collecting your mail.

I had raced through heavy traffic and bad weather to respond to a critical emergency call at the hospital; as I pulled up to the doctors' parking gate, I was already thinking about bypassing the elevators in favor of the back stairway. I was already sorting out different treatment options in my mind. I was trying to picture the patient's face...

As I reached out my car window to punch in the parking lot gate lock code, I had momentary palpitations when I suddenly realized the code didn't work! I damn near broke the gate off after three failed entry tries! Luckily, another doctor showed up and got it to open. I managed to get to the patient in time, but I was not a happy camper.

After an hour of ranting and raving about hospital incompetency, I was politely informed that the doctors' parking lot gate lock code had been changed, and that reminder notices showing the new code had been put in my mailbox every week for the past month...which, of course, I hadn't bothered to check for four to five weeks.

Needless to say, I now make my mailbox a routine checkpoint

with every visit, and arrange for someone on my staff to pick up
my mail when I can't get there.
 — *A red-faced doctor*

The Unbusinesslike Business of Hospital Business

Just as you had never adequately prepared to be a businessperson, and
now — voila — you *are* one, hospitals have never adequately prepared
to be businesses. From their inception, hospitals, like medical practices,
were never intended to be businesses. Yet both are now struggling to
survive as businesses, having been forced to compete as businesses. In
order to survive and compete as businesses, both have absolutely no
choice but to maintain a high level of bottom-line consciousness and a
thorough understanding of what produces profits.

Implied by the use of the word "thorough" is recognition of the fact
that, while turning off office lights, for example, may seem like sound,
economic-minded, profitability sense, it does not increase revenues.
Cutting back marketing programs will save budgeted dollars without a
doubt, but it will cost severely in lost revenue potential and consistency
of image in your internal and external target markets. The only thing that
produces money is sales.

While doctors have generally been savvy enough and financially
capable of hiring top quality businesspeople to surround themselves with
(employees and consultants), hospitals have traditionally lacked both the
awareness and the imagination to look toward business professionals to
guide them. This tends to occur even when the hospital's president, CEO,
CFO, and COO all have solid backgrounds in business.

The result is that most hospitals do recognize that they need sales to
survive and grow, but many of them (as evidenced by massive displays
of fractionalized, inappropriate, uncoordinated, unrealistic, ridiculously
expensive, meaningless marketing programs) haven't a clue about how to
do this. In the event that they are finally able to develop a marketing plan
with impact, it is rarer still that they know how to spend efficiently
whatever dollars they do manage to drum up.

The reluctance or inability of hospital management to pass along
business productivity-oriented thinking to the rank and file has produced
a virtual mountainside of healthcare "sheep" being prodded through
endless mazes of business obstacles by leaders who don't understand why
their people don't take some initiative and risk straying from the herd.

Why don't hospital employees understand? Often, employees are the victims of having been repeatedly slotted into a narrow, dictatorial, vertically-oriented organizational structure that suffocates innovative ideas and actions. It's extremely difficult, for example, to empower employees who have invested in a lifetime of career behavior patterns based on the traditional political framework of a hospital, i.e., a bottom-heavy paternalistic organization where no one wants to make decisions.

Top and (especially) middle management personnel become so dependent on working for "Daddy" (the hospital brass) that they become immobilized and terror-stricken when confronted with the need to take initiative, think and act independently, and/or implement plans of action. Instead, they wait for "Daddy" to approve, direct, order, explain, justify, nurture, and motivate. And "Daddy" waits for them to stop waiting and whining, and start doing. Everybody waits and nothing happens. This vicious cycle of nonactivity undermines both Patient care and doctor relations in "Daddy-directed" organizations.

To make matters worse, many doctors with no other management role models in sight end up adopting the exact same wheel-spinning approach to managing their own practices. Then they wonder why there's no forward movement.

One solo practitioner, age 54, whose frowns, furrowed brow, totally unenergetic voice, and hunched-over posture lead many observers to think he's 104 years old, complains that he is "just plain tired" when asked why he wants to attract a partner or join a group. "Patient flow has slowed down a lot in recent years and I'm growing weary from trying to meet increased expenses. No one in my office seems to have what it takes to help things change. They're all very bright people, but they look to me for the answers on *everything*. They won't buy a box of paper clips without checking with me first. I don't know why, and I don't know how other doctors deal with this, but it looks to me like the hospital has the same problems. I used to think hospital executives had all the answers. I even patterned my business office after the hospital's. I guess times have changed, that's all. I feel old and tired. I hate myself everyday for having become a doctor."

Only a very few hospitals have seen the proverbial light and taken the steps necessary to adapt to the changes being dictated by society and Patient/consumers. Many hospitals, in fearful anticipation of having to become more businesslike, will not survive. Like deer stunned by rapidly approaching headlights, many hospital management teams are poised to die in their tracks. There's no room in today's business world for the inactive. Since the book *In Search of Excellence* by Peters and Waterman

(Harper & Row, New York, 1982) popularized the battle cry, "Do it. Fix it. Try it." as a daily (yea, hourly) method of operation for successful, productive businesses, the awareness has surfaced in literally every top management circle that some action is always better than no action and that when tasks fail to get done by routine methods, try the *un*routine!

The bottom line: If hospitals are to survive, they must change radically. To change radically, they must have your help. They need your active participation in as many different ways as you can possibly afford — policy and procedure recommendation groups, fund-raising committees, community relations programs, in-service training seminars, etc. In case you believe hospital survival isn't important enough to warrant your involvement because you believe independent freestanding facilities (surgi-centers, etc.) can fit the bill just fine, you're wrong. You need these big, inefficient institutions as much as they need you because, as bumbling as they may seem, hospitals remain the best sources of a comprehensive range of specialized healthcare services, equipment, and personnel, the best sources of training, research, and development, and the best sources of public and community relations support. The time to reassess and act on your hospital relationship is now.

While some very few of our country's more progressive hospitals continue to prosper, grow, and serve as guiding lights, most have become too complex, lethargic, unresponsive, undisciplined, insensitive, financially mismanaged, technologically adrift, buried in meaningless paperwork, unsophisticated and outclassed in their marketing, and archaic in their approach to the management of human resources to make a difference in the world, perhaps even to survive, without the input and active support of their physicians.

Setting aside any awareness hospital administrators appear to have of the latest, trendy approaches to management (because that awareness never seems to translate into successful application), hospitals tend to be totally overwhelmed and often without clear definitions of who they are, who their "customers" are, and what their "mission statements" and organizational "visions" are all about.

Hospitals are frequently focused 180 degrees in the wrong direction. Why else is there such insistence that the best parking spaces be allocated to hospital administrators and the "Employee Of The Month?" Whatever privileged parking there is should, if anything, be bestowed on the "Patient of The Month" or "Patient Family of The Month." Why do all the hospital newsletters and news releases highlight hospital accomplishments instead of Patient accomplishments?

These are *not* insignificant points. They are critical representations of misplaced attentions and oblivious, uncaring management. Can you imagine a successful business that allows its employees to park closest to its store or building so that its customers have to hike their way through rows of employee cars to get to the front door? Do hospital administrators think parking lot excursions help Patient visitors (and, thus, Patients) to become less stressed? Isn't the hospital a service-oriented business? Shouldn't the "customer (Patient) always comes first" attitude predominate even more in healthcare than in retail? Surely there are other, more meaningful ways to reward employees beyond spotlighting their good deeds on stages that rightfully belong to Patients and Patient families.

Without a doubt, prospective Patients are more favorably impressed by testimonials from satisfied Patients talking about how great you are than they are by hearing you talk about how great you are. And the same dynamics apply to hospitals, yet hospitals continually chestbeat in their public messages. In many hospitals, entire divisions and departments are so overburdened with outdated organizational structures that they end up defeating their own interests by cultivating work environments, attitudes, and management decision-making that is often only a notch or two above the least efficient of government agencies.

A Conversation in the Hospital Coffee Shop

"Good morning! What can I get for you?"

"Just coffee will be fine, thanks."

"That'll be 39 cents, please."

"Wow. Bargain day, huh?"

"Yeah, it's a lucky thing the hospital owns this business because it would have gone broke a long time ago if it had to be a *real* business."

"What do you mean, it's not profitable?"

"Profitable?! Huh! This place hasn't made a nickel since the day it opened. If they'd let me run it the way I want — with 12 years experience behind me running my father's coffee shop, which was very successful — I'd have this place booming!"

"What happened to your father's place, and what kinds of things would you do here?"

"My dad retired and sold the business to a big chain. And this place here? I'd start by lowering the cost of goods. I'm not allowed to bid out for better quality, less expensive supplies because somebody here is related to somebody in the food company that I have been told to deal with. So, lowering costs for openers. Next, I'd hire some *real* employees to replace the hospital volunteers who don't want to be here in the first place. I would promote with special discount offers to patient visitors, and, in certain cases like maternity, I'd arrange to deliver to rooms so visitors could eat with the patient they're visiting. I would extend the hours the we're open to accommodate evening visitors. I'd run ads in the hospital's publications offering staff discounts during slow times. I would provide 'Emergency Rush' menu items just for doctors by having certain special items that they order most prepared in advance and ready to serve promptly. There's so much that's possible, and they could make a small fortune here if they'd just open their eyes."

"Have you ever suggested taking over the place?"

"No, why bother? Nobody here cares about being like a business. The big shots only worry about fund-raising and contributions and grants and stuff. I hear it all the time when they come in here for coffee. It used to make me crazy; now I just go with the flow. Uh, by the way, how would you like to donate something to our Coffee Shop Capital Improvement Fund?"

Like Jimmy the barber, Stephanie the hairdresser, and Walter the bartender, the hospital coffee shop manager knows almost everything that's going on almost all the time. When you're in doubt about what you hear and can't find the hospital administrator you need to question directly, pay a visit to the coffee shop to enjoy the "view" and see what you learn from listening in on the conversations. A disguised, anonymous visit there will produce an even more realistic view (like the earlier suggestion to pose as a Patient to call your own office) of why nothing in the rest of the world looks or feels the same as it does when you're sitting in the doctor's lounge.

Should Doctors Have Agents?

The idea that doctors, like professional athletes and entertainers, should have agents to represent their interests, negotiate on their behalves with hospitals, and book them into high fee-paying appearances and autograph signings, is fantasy of the highest order (especially the autographs part).

So no agents, right? After all, doctors are not professional athletes. Doctors are not entertainers (although there may be grounds to debate this point in some cases) and doctors are generally better educated than athletes and entertainers, so they can represent their own business interests and negotiate with hospitals for themselves, right? Wrong.

In fact, a "representative" of some kind may, indeed, be appropriate. Many doctors who have turned to management, practice, business, and marketing consultants for help are finding great value. Such consultants can serve as effective translators of the language of "business-ese" and as interpretative resources when it comes to sizing up and evaluating doctor/client concerns, needs, and benefits. They can represent your interests in posturing and communicating with hospitals and other organizational entities. Trusted advisors can also be effective scouts and buffering agents for assessing prospective professional alliances, and for warding off unwanted and persistent sales badgering, especially from potential employees, business suitors, and media representatives.

Consultants will generally have more experience with and a better understanding of organizational dynamics. "Doctors don't understand organizational dynamics," fretted one hospital CEO, "and hospitals are very complex organizations." When asked to elaborate, he said, "Doctors think there's no middle ground on any issue; they think you're either part of the problem or part of the solution. The nature of the beast is that nothing is either black or white, or all or nothing, as most doctors portray. Doctors, don't forget, are trained to be antiauthoritarian and rely only on their own judgements. The fact that so many think that no one can improve on what they have to offer leads a lot of them into extreme behaviors.

"What doctors fail to understand," continued the CEO, "is that while they are trained to do their utmost for every individual case, for every individual patient, as perfectly as humanly possible, it's the job of hospital organizations to do the best we can for the largest numbers of people." He explained that doctors and hospitals have intrinsically adversarial roles, not unlike those that exist for sales and production departments in more traditional companies, where sales people want to speed up production so they can have more inventory available to fill orders, and production people are interested in slowing down production to ensure maximum quality in the units produced.

"Now layer onto the complexity of these reconciliation needs even more complicated doctor/hospital issues...issues such as those involving life and death decisions and actions, tremendous egos, tremendous dollars, women's rights and sexism, and union mentalities that seek to impose seniority-based reward systems over those that encourage and reward performance, and you'll see that the essence of management is discrimination. Doctors don't realize that when you have to deal with more than a three-person staff, things get complex.

"I have a doctor who's been here for 20 years who just told me that 'the hospital is incompetent' because we have 'never done a pelvic prep the right way.' His version of what should be done is different from every other physician's version. Why can't these guys get together and settle on one approach? Instead, they expect us to provide ongoing training and retraining for 400 nurses — not including part-timers and replacements — in each of their individual preferences on how to do a pelvic prep? And what are we supposed to do with all the thousands of other procedures subject to individual doctor preferences?

"Every week, we have to deal with an infuriatingly common (and almost impossible to stop) practice of physicians playing ego/power games with their patients as pawns...'Phantom bookings' are routine, where, for example, a cardiologist can't get catheterizations scheduled when he wants to do them, and so calls with fake bookings for make-believe patient names to block out O.R. time, then switches patients around and changes names...all to suit the doctor's convenience and whimsy. Obviously, this is a more serious problem than overbooking on airlines; this selfish little bit of juggling can easily cost lives. And it is only *not* a problem in those few rare hospitals where doctors value and respect one another."

How does this healthcare leader respond to questions about why hospitals can't simply implement new policies and procedures? "How do you turn a battleship in a narrow, shallow river?" is his answer. It is not so much in mustering the impetus for change, he says, as in "having doctors knock on hospital doors and simply say, 'I want to be part of the solution and I recognize the need to compromise,' and this will only happen when there is trust and respect among doctors."

T.E.A.M. — **Together**
Everyone
Achieves
More
— **U.S. Olympic Gymnastic Champion**
Mary Lou Retton.

XIX

READY, SET...

"Zeal without prudence is like a ship adrift."
— *James Joyce*

When you were learning and training to become a doctor, and again when you started in practice, you undoubtedly had at least some feelings that only a doctoring career could ensure you of personal and professional rewards and satisfaction. Perhaps that same sense of pride and self-confidence still rings true. When did you last measure what you're getting back for what you're giving up?

Stop here for 10 seconds. On a scale of 0 to 10, to what degree is doctoring producing *personal* satisfaction in your life (0 being no satisfaction, 10 being tremendous satisfaction) _____? To what degree is doctoring producing *professional* satisfaction in your life_____? Average satisfaction rating for doctoring in your life overall_____?

If your numbers average out to zero, you should probably consider getting out of the doctoring business. If the numbers average out to anything higher than that, it shows you're still deriving some degree of satisfaction from doctoring, and probably wish you could get more. The only way to achieve higher numbers and more of this highly coveted commodity called "peace of mind" is to adopt a "go with the flow" attitude toward each of life's encounters. This includes encounters with Patients, your family and friends, your financial advisor, your staff members, and your *self*. Expectations breed disappointment. The past is over.

How can you "go with the flow" more than you have been? How can you possibly "go with the flow" when it seems the plumbing is totally clogged up, and there's just a trickle of life managing to seep through the massive rock piles of negativity, anger, resentment, fear, doubt, worry, and guilt?

The Answer

All the tools you could ever need are in this book. But, as with trays full of sterilized equipment, the value of what's put in front of you can only be measured against the potential results when they are used, and when they are used correctly.

If you elect to close or dismiss this book and never review it again, you are passing up your own personal tray of ready instruments. If you decide not to push yourself to do the mental and written exercises this book contains, or if you choose to shut down your receptors and not make continuous efforts to learn more about your *self* and grow your "self" every day, you are choosing the path of self-destruction. If you persist in ignoring the potential of your strengths, and in refusing to address ways to improve your weaknesses; if you do anything short of standing in front of a mirror, looking yourself squarely in the eyes, and vowing to live your life hour by hour with energy, integrity, and sincerity; if you do anything short of using all the self-development instruments put in front of you, you are, in effect, actively choosing for the circumstances of your life to get worse. They surely won't get better. And *nothing* stays the same.

"Honey, I Shrunk My Self!"

With this book, you can increase significantly both revenues *and* Patientflow by using "Quiet Marketing," by reassessing your values, by working to improve your image and your approach, and by freshening up your sense of self-awareness, your goals, your relationship with yourself, and your relationships with others.

With this book, you can "shrink" your *self* by being your own psychologist and your own coach. You can make yourself happier, healthier, and more personally and professionally productive than ever before. It's a choice. It's *your* choice.

Perhaps negative choices you've unwittingly made earlier in your life have accumulated or interacted to the point where the thought of being your own psychologist seems somewhat beyond your grasp. Maybe you don't like probing yourself, or looking at or listening to yourself. Maybe you don't feel confident of being able to produce meaningful results. It could be that you've managed to convince yourself that you're really not ready for this responsibility or that someone else could be a more effective facilitator. If any of these scenarios happens to be the case, then by all means don't try to be your own shrink. Instead, go get one.

If you secretly think you could use a little help, but you feel squeamish, embarrassed, or uncomfortable about exposing your private parts (pardon the double entendre), take heart. You're not by yourself in this respect. Most doctors dislike having to go to other doctors. Even those few doctors who don't hate going to other doctors for physical ailments, usually do hate the idea of anyone "tinkering" with their psyches.

But because you're reading this book, you're smart enough to realize that "psyche tinkering" is hardly representative of what true personal and professional growth and development therapeutic approaches are all about. Squeamishness, embarrassment, and discomfort are unrealistic, fantasized behaviors that are choices. You can *un*choose them, or choose not to have them get in the way of you taking steps on your own behalf. Because you're a doctor, you're smart enough to know that seeing an appropriate psychiatrist, psychologist, therapist, counselor, or personal/professional development coach can most certainly be a "step on your own behalf." The important word here is "appropriate."

"Appropriate" means a professional who encourages you to stay focused on the present; someone who can deliver some immediate insight and results such as help in learning how to deal with your guilt from not having enough time with your family, or from not having been able to save a particular Patient, or in becoming more assertive (or a better listener) in your partner and committee meetings, or in giving up smoking, drinking, gambling, or drugs, or in simply making some immediate changes to live a happier, healthier, more satisfying, more productive life.

Ask around. Check referral services, make some telephone inquiries, ask any friends you know you can trust, or ask some total strangers. If you feel you must give some reason for your shopping survey, respond with "to build my professional referral network." Don't *settle* for anyone, or automatically retain someone's services simply because a friend or colleague gives you glowing reports. Use such recommendations as a starting point, never as a deciding factor. You are *you*, not your friend or colleague. You need to base your decision to see someone not on who recommended them or even whether you *like* that person, but rather on feelings of confidence and trust toward him or her. Otherwise, you cannot expect to experience any decent amount of progress for yourself.

When you do experience the feeling that it's too difficult to step back and examine, treat, motivate yourself, you need to recognize that seeing a psychiatrist, psychologist, therapist, counselor, or personal/professional development coach doesn't make you "a head case," nor is it an incrimination of your sanity. It doesn't mean that anyone who finds out where you're spending your Tuesday nights (or whatever) is going to think you're "loony tunes," or that whoever uncovers or stumbles onto your personal growth and development or problem-solving missions is going to scurry around calling in news reporters for a press conference on your mental and emotional qualifications as a doctor. In fact, anyone who would seek to exploit your self-improvement efforts is someone who truly needs help and (even if it's a partner) should be quickly distanced if that need is not being readily acknowledged.

It makes rational, logical sense to visit with another professional to get help with identifying, sorting out, and evaluating various behavioral options at a time when you've become so overburdened with choices and the accumulation of emotions that your attention easily becomes sidetracked from your family or your practice. Making such visits purely for personal growth and preventive maintenance purposes makes even more sense but, like preventive healthcare visits, is seldom budgeted for or done.

Regardless of your motive, seeing a psychiatrist, psychologist, therapist, counselor, or personal/professional development coach means that you are interested and committed to learning as much as you can about yourself so that you can be even better as a person and as a doctor. It's a way of minimizing and eliminating emotional (and often physical) pain. In the same way an athlete may retain a personal trainer for the purpose of enhancing and peaking personal physical performance levels, engaging a professional for the purpose of enhancing and peaking personal and professional mental/emotional performance levels is a decision that is just plain good sense and well worth the time, expense, and effort involved. This is assuming, as you no doubt have suggested to others, that the prescription is faithfully followed.

Dry Doc

I used to wander the streets aimlessly. I would stare blank stares into blank windows. My only sense of comfort after daily office hours and hospital rounds was in knowing that I had a full flask in my coat pocket, and that I could self-prescribe any mood I felt like being in. I also took some comfort from knowing that no one knew...(every evening it was like having my own private little masturbation session).

My wife ran off with, of all people, a lawyer, and left me alone with two teenagers and the dog. Thank God the kids were fairly self-sufficient! To have only my secret life and coat pocket contents to cling to each night — after spending endless hours listening to other peoples' problems — became disheartening to say the least.

I quickly deteriorated. I kept losing weight. Feeling weak. Shaky. All that candy I'd been eating. Nausea. Sometimes I went for days without shaving or combing my hair. I started wearing sunglasses more. I became afraid to look in the mirror. I feared having to see the sunken, bloodshot, dark-circled eyes that I knew were occupying the top of my face. Looking at a photo someone had taken of me during that time, I could see I had been standing all hunched over; my face was the picture of despair. (It's an absolute wonder that no one caught on. Or maybe someone had. Paranoia. I seemed to be constantly looking over my shoulder when other doctors or nurses were around.)

Then — I can't remember where I was or when — it somehow struck me in one of my sober moments that I should confide in a therapist friend of mine. I guess I had come to the point of thinking that there just wasn't anything else left to happen in my life, except for me to die.

Much to my own amazement, I actually called and made an appointment with my friend. I worried about the risks of talking openly about my secret world, but I was at my wits' end and I could tell that my kids needed more of me than I was able to give. Part of me wanted to run away to some South Sea island. Part of me would have happily settled for the abandoned park bench across from her office. I kept the appointment.

Throughout our first meeting, and for the next two days until I would see her again, she had me do a lot of deep breathing (which I found to be a real struggle...my brain was resisting what my body knew it had to do).

When I returned (a few degrees closer to sober than I had been in many months, but nowhere near where I needed to be), we talked about life being a series of behaviors...and about behavior being a choice...the dim little light bulb I had been carrying around over my head suddenly burst into 1000-watt brightness. I could *choose* to not feel so miserable! How could such a simple thought so ravenously devour my sensibilities?

The realization didn't make me instantly more confident, or provide some miraculous flood of answers. It just gave me a different way of looking at things. I was still filled with doubt, but for the first time in months I felt myself thinking more appreciatively, more positively. I did, after all, still have my two kids...and the dog! I was still a functioning physician and a caring individual. The world had not ended.

Slowly, I began to notice the rumpled, frazzled state of clothes I had been wearing. I overheard two nurses whispering about my disheveledness. I felt embarrassed. I never used to dress that way. I set out to clean up my wardrobe. All by itself, the act of wearing better cared-for clothes led me to the realization that I needed to improve my hygiene — and the food I was eating — pronto!

The food part was easy to decide about, but awfully hard to do. Alcohol can wreak havoc on appetite and taste buds. I knew I wouldn't eat better until I could quit drinking, which I had only managed to slow down a little. Going from a quart of vodka a day to a fifth of vodka a day doesn't make a goddamn bit of difference! It's like cutting back from smoking three packs of cigarettes a day to two and three-quarter packs a day. Big deal!

I couldn't pretend any longer. I enlisted my sister's help to cold turkey the booze. I was lucky. It took me only nine days in the mountains with no flask or refill bottles, no pills, no excuses, lots of exercise and good food (after what seemed like endless vomiting and cramps), and a couple of reinforcement calls to my therapist friend, to completely dry out. At last, I had finally become 'Dry Doc.'

Step at a time, I began to look like a real person again. I began to feel more human too. The challenge, of course, is in being able to stay sober, to stay balanced, to stay above and away from the temptations, to stay alert, to stay in touch with reality, to stay surrounded with supportive, positive people and supportive, positive situations every split second that the option for this choice exists.

Now? I am okay. I did it. I am doing it. I continue, years later, to do it every day, one day at a time. Life is hard enough; going through it in a state of perpetual unconsciousness makes it a hell of a lot harder. But what a battle it was just to realize that all that misery I was mired in was self-created and self-inflicted! This business of 'choosing' and 'choice' might well he the greatest revelation of my life. My rational mind had been so successful at piling up reason upon reason to prevent me from thinking I had any choice about freeing myself from drinking, about freeing myself from negative people and situations, about freeing myself from my own destructive behaviors, from the awareness that I could simply let go...and get on with life.

My story is a good one because I made it through in one piece; with the help of my two rescuers, I survived. Most people who get to where I was, don't make it. Most people don't stop themselves long enough to even think about the fact that (once all the excuses have been set aside), self-destructiveness is a behavior...and behavior is a choice."

That testimony is actually a composite of two separate but almost identical stories recounted by two different doctors at two different times in two different states. Both are now sober — and successful.

Full Circle

Emerging throughout this book is the message that every doctor needs, in varying amounts and frequencies-- to return to some of the basic ideals that prompted pursuit of a doctoring career in the first place. Given the unusually hectic lifestyle most doctors lead, those innocent start-up values can get shoved aside or be completely abandoned within six months of joining or beginning a practice. They can be positively plowed under within five years and rarely ever recalled after a 15-year taste of being on the front lines.

Critical to your ongoing success in the business of your practice, and in the practice of your personal values, is the need to be continually in touch with, and persistently pursuing, those ideas and experiences that lead to newfound levels of self-awareness and to increasing the numbers of "Aha's" of self-discovery in your life. You can only know the candlepower of these enlightenments when you are always seeking and soliciting feedback from others and are continuously conscious of the reality that (actively or inactively, directly or indirectly) you *choose* your own behavior, and that it's just as easy, if not more so, and much more rewarding to choose positive reactions as it is to choose negative reactions!

You also must be constantly taking *action* to combine your increased awareness of your self with your behavioral choices. You must be constantly taking *action* to direct and adjust your own self-management strategies, to lead yourself to enhanced personal and professional growth and development, and to use the tools of personal and professional revitalization that this book has placed in front of you to increase revenues and Patientflow now!

Regardless of anything you read or hear, nothing in the world can be more effective in marketing your doctoring skills than your ability to be ever more authentic in the ways you relate to the rest of the universe, and in your ability to have your sincerity speak for itself.

You need to be aware enough of what's going on in your own office to, for example, respond promptly to another doctor's referral by sending that doctor's *Staff* a six-foot sub sandwich with a "Thank you for referring Mr. Doe to our office" note attached to it. You need to be aware enough of what's going on in your own office to, for example, periodically pass out silver dollars to Staff people you "catch in the act" of smiling or handling a Patient problem positively.

A wonderfully motivating practice that can also have some tangible, clinical value payback (for the increased awareness levels it produces) is to invite nurses and assistants into exam or treatment rooms — whenever it's legal, ethical, and appropriate — to make a point of hosting "on the spot" Patient briefing sessions. This can be done anytime a spare 60 seconds pops up. The bottom line is that the more your people learn, the more helpful they can be to you, and the more professional they can appear, the more they'll appreciate and respect you, and respond positively to you.

Contribute some quality time to a favorite charity or community organization. Carry that "tuned in" level of sensitivity home with you each day. You will become more the very special person you always were meant to be, and the rewards for being that special person will be everlasting. And it's not too late to start "playing music" the minute you put this book down.

...And The Band Played On

Unless you're spending mega-millions for advertising media and agency fees, it's good to remember that advertising is quickly forgotten. Acts of (no cost) genuineness, on the other hand, live on forever in peoples' minds. You're not convinced? Describe the last three advertisements you read or commercials you saw or heard. Include the brand name and any details you can recall. Go ahead. Give it a try:

1)_____

_____

_____

_____

_____

2)_____

_____

_____

_____

_____

3)_____

_____

_____

_____

_____

Now, realizing of course that the probability is you've been exposed to many thousands more advertising messages than acts of kindness, describe (even with that handicap) the last three times someone was especially nice to you:

1)_____

_____

_____

_____

_____

_____

2)_____

_____

_____

_____

_____

_____

3)_____

_____

_____

_____

_____

_____

How would you sum up in one or two words your recollection of the first three "messages?"

1)_____

2)_____

3)_____

How would you sum up in one or two words your recollection of the second set of "messages?"

1)_____

2)_____

3)_____

Which had more impact?
☐ Advertising Messages   ☐ Behavior Messages   ☐ No Difference

Which would most prompt you to tell others about what you recall?
☐ Advertising Messages ☐ Behavior Messages ☐ No Difference

Considering that you are exposed to roughly 2,500 advertising messages a *day* (even if you don't watch TV), how significant do you think this little itemization above really is? Can you apply anything you might learn (from thinking about this exercise) to your own personal approach to marketing your practice? What specific thoughts come to mind?

_____

_____

_____

_____

_____

_____

_____

_____

_____

_____

Ha, Ha, Ha, Ha, Ha, Ha, Ha!

"Where laughter fails to heal, it never fails to ease the pain."
— *A terminal cancer Patient*

Nothing heals or binds people together like laughter, the magic ingredient that's highly prevalent in successful Patients, practices, organizations, marriages, families, and partnerships. Laughter is a universal symbol of mental and emotional health. Mental and emotional health is increasingly being credited by leading, proactive, Patient-centered care organizations and individuals as a key source of physical health. For numerous, clear references that underscore this emerging consciousness, read Bill Moyers' *Healing And The Mind* (Doubleday, New York, 1993). Many of Moyers' interview subjects, including prominent medical doctors, support the estimate that mental and emotional health accounts for major portions, if not all, of physical health. Regardless of the degree of impact of psychoimmunology, there is clearly no longer any dissention among professionals that mental and emotional wellness and the positive attitudes that accompany it can go a long way toward mending, healing and restoring physical health.

Did you get the last laugh when you last laughed, or were you simply laughing to enjoy the spirit of the moment? Come to think of it, *when* did you last laugh? If you might generally measure the answer to this question in minutes, you're probably a high-spirited, high energy level, positive attitude, productive-type individual (or an actor). If you would tend to measure your response in terms of hours, you're probably ahead of the (doctor) pack, but not by much. If you can only answer the question in numbers of days or weeks, you clearly need more humor in your life, and you probably shouldn't wait for longer than it takes to finish reading this page to do or say or think something funny. Even watching some "no-brainer" television sitcom is better than nothing. Nothing begets nothing.

When did you last *hug*? Family therapist and author Virginia Satir says it takes 12 hugs a day to grow. What does your scorecard look like for today? Yesterday? Was your last hug one that *you* initiated, one that was delivered *to* you, or a spontaneous mutual event? Was it a real hug or a token hug? (You know the token ones. Those are where little more than cheeks, maybe shoulders, and possibly a tiny hunk of chest actually touch.) These hugs are usually accompanied by a forced smile and some ridiculously meaningless words of phoney admiration, half whispered into your hair or sideburns, such as, "So nice to see you again, dear," and "You're looking as lovely as always, darling." There are also token bear hugs. These come along every once in awhile from some well-intentioned oaf who really never learned how to hug. You usually can tell when you're getting one of these hugs when your feet start to lift off the ground and you can't get your hands out of your pockets!

When did you last pat someone on the back for a job well done? A Patient's back? A parent's back? A child's back? A spouse or significant other's back? A Staff member's back? Another doctor's back? How about your own back? Doctors who make a practice of dispensing these pats (warmly and genuinely), whenever their hands are free, are writing their own referral tickets. People appreciate being appreciated, especially for doing small deeds and accomplishing routine little tasks that ordinarily go unnoticed.

When did you last smile in the mirror and really mean it? If it wasn't this morning, you may need to start liking yourself more. It's not such a difficult challenge. You have an awful lot of good qualities, and every day is a great opportunity to be the best that you can be. It's also terribly difficult to appreciate and love others when you don't appreciate and love yourself.

When did you last say "I love you"? Motivational speaker and author Zig Ziglar says you should try to absolutely bowl over your spouse with affection every night. Take the risk of utter shock by doing it every night for a week and see the results. You might even experience immediate returns! Just free yourself to say how truly appreciative you are for your husband or wife or lover's existence, and for all the little things you never acknowledge that make life worth living and that help you to be more of the person you want to be, the person you are becoming.

"Thank you for helping me become the person I am" or "Thank you for helping me become a more authentic person" or "Thank you for helping me to grow" or "Thank you for being such a positive influence in my life" or "Thank you for being so supportive when I needed it" are all wonderful statements that set off lots of little explosions of happiness and good feelings when they're expressed sincerely. Wouldn't you like hearing comments like these yourself?

"I will take care of me for you
if you will please take care of you for me."
— Anonymous

XX

...GO!

It makes no difference whatsoever what launch pad you're poised on, whether you're affiliated with one or more HMO's, PPO's, EPO's, IPA's, PHO's, Individual Practices, Group Practices, Network Practices, or Hospital-Based Practices, and regardless of whether you function on a capitation or fee-for-service system; when you ignite this book's principles, you will blast off into increased revenue and Patient flow orbits.

It is important that you refocus your thinking and erase your preconceived notions about what "marketing" is *supposed* to be. Stop listening to cocktail party and family gathering gibberish about vertical and horizontal markets, reach and frequency, SOM (share of market) determinants, CPM's (cost per thousand, a reference to advertising media expenses relative to numbers of audience reached), subliminal messages, and overexposed spokespersons.

Stop thinking there's some glamorous association between this foreign world of business marketing and your practice pursuits. There's not. When conversations turn in these directions, you can be interested, but you will probably accomplish more in the way of marketing your practice by excusing yourself to study the room's paint job or corner molding, or by stepping outside to contemplate the name "Bandurski" on the neighbor's mailbox.

You need to zero in on the reality that the only avenue to true (financial and psychic reward-filled) professional success is the personal avenue within yourself, the one which connects your thoughts and feelings with your behaviors.

You need to reject all the textbook and big business ideas and hype about media and creative plans and approaches. Put all the notions aside that suggest you should be concentrating on ways to implement or strengthen your efforts in selling, advertising, promotion, public relations, direct mail, coupons, telemarketing, merchandising, et al. These are only secondary, supportive, reflective tools. They cannot stand on their own.

Instead of reflecting on these concepts, snap your fingers or whistle or clap your hands or slap your thighs to bring your brain back into reality, and accept the fact that the marketing approach that's the most effective, most pervasive, most persuasive, and has the highest impact imaginable for any doctor or healthcare practice will be, in reality, one that originates and maintains itself "quietly, from within." It is with this understanding, and with purposeful forward movement toward developing and consistently nurturing these "Quiet Marketing"-based values, messages, and methods, that you can actually propel yourself to within reaching distance of realizing your dreams — for your Patients, your practice, your family, and yourself.

This is not to suggest that you abandon the basics or ignore what you know to be effective. Don't suddenly discard the marketing you've already been using, especially if it's working. Above all, you will want to be sure you're at least doing the following:

• You still need to define clearly the exact segment of the healthcare and geographic market you most want to carve out for yourself. Given a range of factors that include your expertise, training, experience, interests, market density and composition, intra-doctor and community politics, hospital politics, referral network potential, number and strength of directly competitive practices, etc., pick the one target market that has the best odds for success. Do *not* select the one that represents the greatest challenge, or that's untried and unproven. Leave these high-risk expeditions for the fearless explorers who have plenty of fortitude and *plenty* of cash.

• You still need to have a basic practice brochure, folder, or booklet that outlines your practice's policies and procedures, your personal and professional training, experience, any special skills or interests, and a professionally-taken photo of your cheerful, friendly-looking self. (No matter how serious your personality or specialty may be, there's no need to represent yourself or your practice in somber, funereal tones. Don't give people even more reason to worry than they already have, unless you're drumming up enrollments for a friend's stress management course.)

• You still need to have established systems and methods for channeling your (nonPatient exam and treatment) energy and time into building and maintaining solid rapport with referral bases, solid, long-term relationships with networks and individuals.

• You still must make a habit of being constantly alert to ways of improving your scheduling efficiency. You must follow up tenaciously with every reasonable possibility.

• You still need to be giving as many talks, seminars, and presentations as you can comfortably accommodate in your life.

• You still need to be a perpetual student of your specialty or special areas of interest. You cannot know too much about health, healthcare, and wellness.

When you're developing and activating these essential "Quiet Marketing" ingredients, remember that the one that is most essential because it single-handedly protects all the others, is to do your own primary care on your *self*!

You must work at letting go of some those protective layers of secrecy and security you've wrapped around your ego. You must be willing and committed to work relentlessly, with almost reckless abandon, to make everything you do as personalized as possible to those you do things for. The more you go to great lengths to treat others the ways you want most to be treated yourself, the closer you get to becoming the doctor you have always known you were capable of becoming.

Whether you've been in practice for 30 or 40 years or you're a first-year student, and no matter what type of doctor you are, you no doubt know that "being a doctor" and "practicing medicine" (or "healthcare") are entirely different states of mind. Anyone who does the necessary studying and passes the necessary tests can earn a "doctor" title. It takes the very special person that you have the potential to be even more of, to *be* a doctor.

Every time you notice one of those daytime processions of cars with their headlights on passing you on the road, be reminded of your own human frailty. Be reminded that happiness is the way. Be reminded that you become what you think about. Remember that deep breathing soothes your neurological system, relaxes your muscles, and makes your brain more alert. The easiest and best solution to any problem lies within the individual (or group) who (that) has the problem. When two children (or partners) are arguing over a piece of cake (or a policy, procedure, or benefit), the response that's always proven most effective is to designate one to "slice" it and the other to have first choice.

Above all else, your genuine success can only come from your genuine love of your self, of your family and friends, of your Staff and associates, of your Patients, of what you do, and of who you are becoming. Every hour. Every day. Every night.

Eight last "food for thought questions" as you complete *Doctor Business* and begin the first day of your next journey:

• How much easier is it now (or, at least, how much more conscious are you of the need) to stop "playing the role" of doctor, and start "being" a doctor (as compared with when you first started reading this book)? Can you start "being" a doctor the minute you close this book's cover?

• How much will your own increased emphasis on authenticity help you to be a better professional, and a better person? Can you start being more authentic the minute you close this book's cover?

• What do you imagine your practicing higher levels of authenticity can produce for you in terms of revenues and Patientflow? Can you make a guess and set a goal about this *before* you close this book's cover?

• How can being more authentic help you keep your personal life together along the way? Can you start collecting and connecting your personal life more effectively and with more meaning the minute you close this book's cover?

On your way to becoming the very best you can be, get in the habit of making something wonderful happen each day before you sleep — like right *now*. No excuses. What were you planning to do when you finished this book anyway? Take an extra minute. Think of some outstanding, happy thing you could do or say that could make the whole day a great one for yourself and/or someone else; some words or action that will make you grin as your head hits the pillow tonight. Crank up an extra splash of energy from deep inside. Then, as a popular advertising message suggests, *Just Do It!*

If you already did do something wonderful today, then go right ahead and get that elusive night's sleep you so richly deserve. You're definitely going to need it. Why? Because when you wake up tomorrow, you will be facing the greatest opportunity of your entire life.

****

Your inquiries, thoughts, success stories and responses to *Doctor Business* are always welcome to be considered for incorporation into future editions. All communications will be treated confidentially and answered personally by the author.

To arrange customized organizational or practice development consulting with the author, or schedule a group presentation, you may contact him directly at:

BUSINESSWORKS
Consultants To The Health Professions
MidLantic Bank Plaza
1091 River Avenue
Lakewood, NJ 08701
Phone: 908/901-7353
Fax: 908/901-0770

****